Values-Based Interprofessional Collaborative Practice

Working Together in Health Care

Jill E. Thistlethwaite

Professor of Medical Education and Director,
Centre for Medical Education Research and Scholarship,
School of Medicine, University of Queensland,
Australia

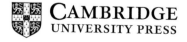

CAMBRIDGE
UNIVERSITY PRESS

CAMBRIDGE UNIVERSITY PRESS
Cambridge, New York, Melbourne, Madrid, Cape Town,
Singapore, São Paulo, Delhi, Mexico City

Cambridge University Press
The Edinburgh Building, Cambridge CB2 8RU, UK

Published in the United States of America by Cambridge University
Press, New York

www.cambridge.org
Information on this title: www.cambridge.org/9781107636163

First published 2012

Printed and bound in the United Kingdom by the MPG
Books Group

*A catalogue record for this publication is available from the
British Library*

Library of Congress Cataloguing in Publication data
Thistlethwaite, Jill.
Values-based interprofessional collaborative practice : working
together in health care / Jill E. Thistlethwaite.
p. ; cm.
Includes bibliographical references and index.
ISBN 978-1-107-63616-3 (pbk.)
I. Title.
[DNLM: 1. Patient Care Team.   2. Community Networks.
3. Interprofessional Relations.   4. Patient Care – ethics.
5. Professional Practice – ethics.   W 84.8]
610.73 – dc23   2012021825

ISBN 978-1-107-63616-3 Paperback

Contents

Preface

This book is one of a series on values-based practice (VBP). It has a specific focus on teamwork and collaborative health care practice particularly, but not exclusively, in primary care. The health care teams considered include nurses (practice and advance practitioners), midwives, general practitioners (GPs) and hospital doctors, physiotherapists and other allied health professionals as well as receptionists and practice managers. The book considers the interactions between health care professionals and the way that these may be affected by differences in professional and personal values, amongst other factors. The scenarios are informed by my experience in general practice in both the UK and Australia, but they can be adapted to family medicine situations in other countries.

This book is thus for all health care professionals who work in teams or aspire to collaborative practice, and for educators who facilitate learners in teamwork. Health professional students should also find it useful and hopefully stimulating, while the scenarios may be helpful for learning activities.

The text contributes to the literature on consultation and communication skills by adding the dimension of values-based practice, which is rarely mentioned in other work of this nature. It is a practical guide, underpinned by theory, to health care interactions. The underlying philosophy of values-based practice, as described and discussed by my colleagues, Professors Bill Fulford and Ed Peile, in their own work, will be the starting point for the text. However I also consider and reflect on working in teams and the importance of communication.

Health and social care within the NHS in the UK is now largely team based; from the primary care team of community settings to the multidisciplinary teams of secondary care, as particularly exemplified by cancer and diabetes management. The ageing population and the rise in the incidence of long term chronic and complex conditions mean that one health care professional is unlikely to have the knowledge and skills to provide complete care. The growing team work literature highlights the difficulties of diverse professionals coming together to work together with their unique professional identities, their changing roles and responsibilities and, for many, their lack of training in team work at prequalification level. Add to this both personal and professional values bases, and we can see that communication is fraught with difficulty. Poor communication is implicated as a major cause of adverse events in health care and leads to poor patient safety. Lack of communication between professionals and dysfunctional teamwork have been repeatedly shown to contribute to poor patient and client outcomes.

Why a values-based approach?

Health care practitioners from different professional backgrounds may work together in defined co-located teams or collaborate across sites to achieve specific goals over a limited time frame. Not all professionals interacting with the same patient are members of the same team – some provide a limited amount of input in highly specialised areas. To provide such collaboration and, where relevant, team-based care, there is a necessity not only to learn the appropriate skills but also to explore and understand each other's values, and those of the people we care for and treat.

If health professionals have competing values, arising from their professional identity and/or cultural background and/or personal experiences, there is likely to be miscommunication. In my experience health professionals rarely put aside time to discuss their values with their colleagues, though some may adopt a values-based approach with patients/clients. Stereotyping of professionals by professionals occurs frequently, e.g., the arrogant doctor, the caring nurse, the efficient pharmacist. In this book I consider how professionals may discuss their values – through learning together and working together.

My experience

I bring to this volume my own experience of interprofessional education (IPE) and collaborative practice, my 26 years as a practising general practitioner (GP) and my 22 years as a clinical educator. As a young GP principal in West Yorkshire I was fortunate to be a member of a highly developed primary care team and valued the interactions with other health professionals from which I learnt a great deal. The team included practice and district nurses, health visitors, psychologists and physiotherapists, and community midwives who worked with the doctors to provide high quality antenatal and post-natal care, plus home and hospital births. As well as the health professionals, the receptionists and secretaries were indispensible. We had the usual problems of arguments about workload and pay, but were united in aiming to provide the best care for our patients. In my early career I tended to be paternalistic towards patients, a consequence of my hospital training, but I discovered the concepts of shared decision making and moved towards a more patient partnership model.

I don't remember an explicit discussion about practice values but we had a 'mission statement' and regular team meetings for both business and education. This teamwork aspect of my work was what I missed most when I moved to Australia and worked as a sessional GP while pursuing my career as an academic medical educator. My experience is that teamwork and collaborative practice are very variable in their quality depending on the people involved, their values and commitment to health care delivery. My involvement in the teaching of communication and consultation skills over the years has shown me that performance may be improved but that it is important to involve a range of health professionals in learning together to break down existing stereotyping and the hierarchical nature of some clinical environments.

I must emphasise that as a medical doctor I have a certain view of health care practice. I have tried to think from the perspective of other professionals and patients in this work and have had both feedback on the text and input to some chapters as commentaries from colleagues and service users. However if it feels too medical I do apologise. Mostly I use the word patient, but I acknowledge that others may refer instead to client, service user or consumer.

Overall structure of the book

The opening chapters include an overview of values-based practice, teamwork and collaborative practice to set the scene for the subsequent case histories. After the introductory chapters, subsequent chapters present case histories and scenarios based on authentic professional experiences with details changed to preserve confidentiality. The scenario generates reflection points and readers are encouraged to stop and reflect where indicated. Selected chapters have comments from patients and appropriate health care professionals to add different perspectives. I use relevant references to provide evidence for certain statements and to indicate the range of literature on particular topics. There are concluding chapters on learning and teaching in this area. While the book predominantly focuses on teams and health care delivery in primary care settings and general practices (because of my experience), there are references to hospital-based and secondary care settings as well.

Synopsis of the chapters

Chapter 1: Values-based practice in health care: setting the scene

This chapter includes an overview of VBP with definitions of values and a discussion about their diversity. I consider value judgments, personal and professional values and the hidden curriculum. VBP and evidence-based practice are compared, and I look at the barriers to VBP.

Chapter 2: Teamwork and collaborative practice in modern health care

Here I consider the concept and practice of teamwork and its relationship to collaborative practice. There are definitions of team and how teams function, and of the meaning of interprofessional in this context. I discuss how team members may have different values and why it is important that teams reflect both on the team's and the members' values. There is a section on the competencies required for collaborative practice and the barriers that include professional stereotyping.

Chapter 3: Communication within teams and between professionals

In this chapter I consider the evidence about the importance of good communication for patient outcomes and safety, including communication via team meetings and medical records. The scenario is based on an interaction involving a GP, a nurse, a receptionist and a patient during which the wrong injection is given. High expectations, including the need to be perfect, by one member of the team may cause repercussions if others cannot meet these high standards. Professionals need to be able to delegate and handover needs to be undertaken carefully. Constructive feedback is important when dealing with interpersonal issues and conflict.

Chapter 4: A patient complaint: team meetings, policy and practice values – raising awareness in the team

Using the scenario of a patient complaint as the basis for discussion, I consider in further detail the importance of team meetings and record keeping, as well as significant event analysis (SEA) and the concept of health literacy. This chapter finishes with a lay commentary.

Chapter 5: A well person check, health promotion and disease prevention: different lifestyles, different values

What does being healthy mean to people and what is the value of health checks? There may be a difference of opinion amongst the health professionals about health, preventing illness and screening. I discuss evidence-based practice and how evidence changes and is interpreted. How professionals work together to manage patients with chronic disease is an important focus of the chapter.

Chapter 6: A patient with medically unexplained symptoms: applying evidence and values for shared decision-making, self-care and co-production of health

Patients who present with multiple symptoms and no clear diagnosis are a challenge for all team members. It is important that patients receive a clear and consistent message from the professionals with whom they interact. I stress that these are not difficult patients but difficult consultations.

Chapter 7: A request for strong analgesia: honesty and trust

Honesty and trust are two values required for good working relationships. Interactions between patient and professional as well as between professionals are difficult without being able to assume honesty. The scenario considers what may be an inappropriate request for strong painkillers and how the team may deal with the issue. How is trust built and maintained?

Chapter 8: Asylum seekers and refugees: working across cultures

The case of an asylum seeker is the stimulus for discussing culture, prejudice and racism. I revisit health literacy and discuss the concept of cultural sensitivity. Health professionals also come from diverse countries and cultures, which affects their values and practice. We conclude with considering training to overcome racial prejudice and the challenges of working with interpreters.

Chapter 9: A request for a home birth and other pregnancy-related consultations

This chapter looks at patient options and shared decision making through scenarios focusing on pregnancy and giving birth. A midwife colleague provides a concluding section – giving a different professional perspective.

Chapter 10: Community-based care and the wider health team

This chapter has been written by Dawn Forman, a radiographer by initial training, and now professor of interprofessional education at Curtin University (Australia). Dawn considers the wider health care team in a scenario in which one partner of a married couple is moved into a residential care home. She explores how team-based care may be improved. The case study can be used to stimulate discussion of the patient and client needs in a care environment.

Chapter 11: Ageing and end of life decisions

End of life care is a very challenging, but rewarding, area for the health care team. There are ethical and values-based considerations, and potentially very diverse opinions amongst team members. I consider advance directives/decisions, euthanasia and assisted suicide as areas where values may conflict. The chapter concludes with comments from a nursing and education colleague, who researches into end of life care.

Chapter 12: Referrals and the interface between primary and secondary care: looking after 'our' patients

Patients are cared for in both primary and secondary care settings. In this chapter I discuss the issues relating to referral from one team to another, difficulties with care across the primary secondary care interface, and how teams function in hospitals. The implications of defining someone as 'my' patient are discussed. The chapter concludes with a patient's perspective.

Chapter 13: Living with visible difference and valuing appearance

This chapter considers the modern fixation with appearance and the concept of visible difference. There are many examples of value judgments relating to how we look including size, 'beauty' and scarring. One section of the chapter is written by a lay colleague.

Chapter 14: Collaboration with other professionals: in and outside health care

What about working with pharmacists, social workers, the police and teachers? These professionals are not usually members of the team but part of our wider collaboration.

Chapter 15: Learning in and about teams

Here I focus on how teams can learn together to work together, including through role-play and working with simulated patients. Interprofessional education is a key requirement for collaborative practice.

Ways of using this book

This will very much depend on the reader and previous knowledge/experience of teamwork and/or values-based practice. Someone fairly new to the topics would be advised to start with the introductory section to understand the concepts. Educators or more experienced professionals may dip into a particular scenario to begin with – one that resonates with their own practice and that may also be useful for discussion as a learning activity. They could then read other chapters that interest them, while referring back to part 1 to revise their knowledge and/or to gain a better understanding of the messages and reflections in the scenarios.

Acknowledgements

I would like to thank Professor Bill Fulford for inviting me to write this book and for his clarification of how values-based practice complements my thinking on consultation skills and interprofessional practice.

My interprofessional mentors include Emeritus Professors Hugh Barr (UK) and John Gilbert (Canada) in addition to my interprofessional colleagues around the world for their insights into and commitment to IPE, which can be challenging in the face of logistics and frequent negativity.

Specific thanks to Krysia Saul, Sally Brown, Judy Purkis, Ann Jackson and Dawn Forman for their contributions to the chapters.

I have learnt most from 'my' patients over the years: I would not be the doctor today who listens without their feedback. I acknowledge our partnerships and the teams in which I have worked.

Last but not least, I thank my partner George Ridgway for his support, patience and numerous re-locations over the years.

Forewords

We value or devalue other professions in the adjectives that we employ to describe them, and the stereotypes to which we resort, as contributors to this book will have been well aware. Readers and writers alike, we are all products of professionalisation, a process as subtle as it can be subversive when it invites invidious comparisons between 'them' and 'us'. Explanations for the relative value that we accord the professions are as many as they are varied. They are rooted in gender, social class, schooling and subsequent professional education, including the relative status of the universities in which it is provided, in the length of their courses, in the level of their awards, in the emphases in curricula on the sciences and the humanities and on specialist and generalist practice.

Differences such as these are diminishing in country after country. The number of men and women entering the health professions is becoming more evenly balanced. Doors are opening for students from disadvantaged backgrounds to enter the more prestigious professions via access programmes. Profession-specific colleges are being merged into the newer universities which are closing the academic gap with the older universities. Professional awards are evening up as more professions establish graduate entry and marriages are made between scientific and humanitarian curricula.

Yet prejudice persists between professions. Educational engineering is not enough; interprofessional education makes good the shortfall. It provides a level playing field for the learners, where the centre forward is neither more nor less valued than the half back or the goalkeeper. It creates opportunities where students entering each of the health professions learn to rely on the others as together they appraise the values, insights and expertise that each brings to perform its allotted role, relinquishing preconceptions and stereotypes when necessary.

Professionalism is enhanced; positive values of interdependence and collective responsibility wax as negative values of sectional interest wane. Boundaries become permeable in the age of open communication and the liberation of knowledge, as roles and relationships are redefined. The value of each profession is enhanced by the esteem which it comes to enjoy not only in the eyes of other professions but also of patients, public and policy makers as it responds more readily and more effectively to their competing expectations in a spirit of closer collaboration.

Where better to begin to reflect on the values that permeate personal, professional and interprofessional practice with clients and colleagues?

Hugh Barr
Emeritus Professor of Interprofessional Education and Honorary Fellow
University of Westminster, UK
President, Centre for the Advancement of Interprofessional Education (CAIPE)

Educators of health care professionals, both those who work on university and college campuses, and those who provide learning environments in practice settings, are increasingly expected to understand and develop collaborative team based scenarios. Over the past 50 years, our understanding of 'health', and the complexities of providing the highest quality of care, has forced a radical rethink of the spectrum of education necessary for competent and efficient practice.

The task of understanding "the team" as a flexible unit of work has been greatly enhanced by research in organisational psychology, and other related social sciences. Bringing this work to the notice of those in health professional education is one of the major functions of this book. As both a monograph and a textbook, it uses logic derived from practice in primary care to the construction of relevant scenarios that illustrate ways and means of "experiencing" the complex interactions between a variety of health professionals, which are the basis of high functioning teams.

Two major issues confront the development of such teams: trust and information transfer (all too frequently referred to as communication). This book treats both matters in detail and frames them within the context of values-based practice – a context that is woefully lacking (and sometimes lost) in discussions about evidence-based practice.

Interprofessional education for collaborative patient-centred practice and care is the ideal focus of this book, although not its only intended aim. As health care systems throughout the world continue to grapple with how best to construct primary health care systems that hold true to the ideal of the WHO Alma-Ata Declaration of 1978, this book has some forceful insights to offer from the author's practice. The complexities of "communication" are presented within the context of scenarios that make plain the fact that "communication" is not simply about polite enquiry. Various investigations of adverse events underline the immense importance of not only using the right words, but also of using the words right!

At base, the differences between health professionals are in many ways attributable to differences in values that profoundly affect their behaviour. This book deals clearly with these difficult and contentious matters in ways that illustrate the differences without assigning blame. The author recognizes that all health professionals come from somewhere, and that regardless of work setting, they are inevitably situated within their personal culture – the place of a lifetime of learning; that their daily motivation to action is guided by their personal culture and that their interaction with others in daily practice is inevitably bound to their individual cultural understanding. This book deals sensitively and wisely with these issues, and presents the reader with many opportunities to test her/his perceptions against the realities of practice as illustrated in the scenarios.

This is not a book for the faint-hearted! Tough questions are posed, and challenging suggestions made. If (and at this time the "if" is very large) our health care system is to change, then the education of health care professionals, in all its environments, must inevitably start the journey to learn "with, from and about each other, for the purposes of collaboration to improve the quality of care" (CAIPE 2002 and WHO 2010) as soon as possible, or sooner! This book provides an intriguing and important place from which to start that journey.

John H.V. Gilbert, C.M., Ph.D., FCAHS
Principal & Professor Emeritus, College of Health Disciplines
University of British Columbia

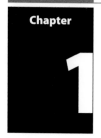

Values-based practice in health care: setting the scene

'If there is any merit in this idea at all, the VDM (values-based decision making) offers a hugely exciting prospect for greater tolerance and understanding between human beings.'
(Seedhouse, 2005, page 47)

Values-based health and social care practice is an approach that aims to involve both patient and professional in decision making and management, taking into account both parties' views. It may be seen as complementary to what are claimed as the more scientific aims of evidence-based practice, which some practitioners and patients consider has reduced rather than enhanced the possibility of patient partnership. There is an emphasis in the health professional literature, particularly from medicine, on evidence-based practice often without a mention of values. In this chapter I will explore the nature of both values-based and evidence-based practice in general, while chapter 2 considers values as they affect teamwork and collaborative practice.

Definitions of values

One definition of values is that they 'operate as standards by which our actions are selected' (Mason et al., 2010, page 71). Also succinctly 'a value is a belief upon which man acts by preference' (Allport, 1961, page 454). In relation to patients, values are 'the unique preferences, concerns and expectations each patient brings to a clinical encounter and which must be integrated into clinical decisions if they are to serve the patient' (Thornton, 2006, page 2). Fulford et al. (2012), in the first volume of this series, use the term 'values' to include 'anything positively or negatively weighted as a guide to health care decision-making'. Values-based care or values-based practice (VBP) similarly has a number of definitions (Box 1.1).

Many of the definitions arise from work involving mental health services. For example the National Institute for Mental Health in England (NIMHE – now known as the National Mental Health Development Unit NMHDU) has developed a national framework of values for mental health, guided by three key principles of values-based practice. These principles are recognition, raising awareness and respect for diversity. The framework stresses that values as well as evidence must be recognised as having a role in mental health policy and practice. Professionals need to be aware of differences in values and how these may affect their practice in mental health. This diversity should be respected to ensure not only equality but to avoid discrimination for any reason such as age, gender, cultural background, sexuality, religion or

Box 1.1: Definitions of values-based practice

'…a blending of the values of both the service user and the health and social care professional, thus creating a true, as opposed to a tokenistic partnership' (Thomas et al., 2010, page 15).

'The theory and capabilities for effective decision making in health and social care that builds in a positive way on differences and diversity of values' (University of Lincoln, online).

Fulford et al. (2012), in the first volume of this series, define values-based practice as consisting of a premise, process and point. Starting from the 'democratic' premise of mutual respect for differences of values, they describe a 10-part process to achieve the 'point' of balanced decision-making within frameworks of shared values.

race. Respect for values is a reciprocal process: the patient and all involved in care including the different professionals, carers and health services have to be aware of and respond to values, taking them into account in diagnosis, management and follow-up.

The importance of VBP has been recognised by its inclusion as part of the UK Royal College of General Practitioners' (RCGP) curriculum for British general practitioners. This states that all GPs should be able 'to understand the nature of values and how these impact on healthcare' (RCGP, online). Moreover, GPs should be able to 'recognise their personal values and how these affect their decision-making'.

Reflection point

If you are new to the concept of values, or haven't really thought about your own definition, pause to consider what you and other people might mean by 'my values'.

You will probably use some of the following words and terms: principles, beliefs, ethics, standards, conscience, virtues.

A value can be a belief, a mission, a motivating force, an ideal or a philosophy that has meaning for an individual, community or organisation. An individual may not be aware of holding, choosing or developing these values until challenged, or put into a situation where others have different or opposing values, leading to potential conflict. When asked to define your own values, you may also include words or terms that refer to some of the actual values that you do hold: being fair, telling the truth, kindness, respect, obeying the law, being a hard worker, helping people less fortunate than yourself, altruism, integrity, loyalty, self-reliance, putting family first. You may think of professional values such as being punctual, being smartly dressed, being a good communicator, not breaking confidentiality, putting the patient first, going that extra mile for the patient or community; all very positive. But your value-system might also include a darker side: making sure you get your rights, aiming to be better than others, striving to come top of the class, doing whatever it takes to succeed. I have labelled these 'darker' but that is my value judgment and certainly not everybody's.

The diversity of values

If you now ask the question, what do I value most in life, your list may include other items such as: my family, my health, job, colleagues, religion, car, exotic holidays etc. This shows the power of one English word and the connotations it can hold. Value, and its adjective valuable, is also used to mean monetary worth, though something may have sentimental value to one person, while being worthless to another. In certain societies everything may have a price: loyalty, affection, trust, until a higher bidder comes along and there is a transfer of such attributes for greater profits. Thus saying that something is valuable to me has little meaning unless the context is clear. I may say to a colleague 'I value your opinion' until I hear what that opinion is and belittle it, negating my previous statement and showing that I only value their opinion if it resonates with my own. On the other hand I may listen to their opinion and find it very useful.

A group of people that looks homogeneous from the outside may be made up of individuals with very different values. We often assume that people we like, we work with, who are on our team, who are in the same profession, whom we respect, have similar values to our own, but it is not something we usually explore when making acquaintances, or working with new colleagues or when we join a new team: we usually pick up on their values in our interactions, and they pick up on ours.

The Australian Government Department of Immigration and Citizenship gives a list of Australian values that I had to commit to when becoming an Australian citizen (Box 1.2).

Box 1.2: Values of Australian citizens (Australian Government, 2011)

- Respect for the freedom and dignity of the individual
- Equality of men and women
- Freedom of religion
- Commitment to the rule of law
- Parliamentary democracy
- A spirit of egalitarianism that embraces mutual respect, tolerance, fair play and compassion for those in need and pursuit of the public good
- Equality of opportunity for individuals, regardless of their race, religion or ethnic background.

The department goes on to state that 'although these values may be expressed differently by different people, their meaning stays the same. The values may not be unique to Australia, but they have broad community agreement and underpin Australian society and culture'. Apart from parliamentary democracy being irrelevant in the health context, there is probably nothing here that a health professional would disagree with, but there could be conflicts with others in the way we interpret the values and there are other values that might also underpin our work.

We make value judgments every day: from the mundane (is this computer worth this much to me?) to more important decisions which may have profound effects (can I trust this doctor? Can I trust this health professional? Can this patient make an informed consent?) When considering such judgments, we need to have a choice of behaviour. If there is only one option, there is nothing to judge, unless there is the option to do nothing.

How do we know what our values are? How do we develop or acquire our values? We acquire our personal values early in life and develop them as we mature; they shape and influence how we think and what we do (Warne & McAndrew, 2008). We may not be aware of them until we are tested. Mason et al. (2010) have suggested that 'identifying one's values requires a person to decisively penetrate their moral index and form a values inventory' while stating that 'in reality, most people are living the values of others' (page 73).

We may think we hold values but we may soon lose some of these when tested (as before: everything has a price). I may hold the value that stealing is wrong, but not speak up if given too much change when shopping, or not declare that extra bit of untaxed income to the Inland Revenue. In the latter case, my value of honesty is outweighed by my belief that it is perfectly ok to try to pay less tax using any means possible.

Most of the time we are not aware of our values in our choices, but when we are faced with conflicting values we may become uneasy, and decisions are likely to be more difficult. There may be conflicts between our own values, or between our values and others we interact with. For example, a health practitioner's professional values may include thinking that using marijuana is wrong as it is illegal and harmful; however his personal values based on experience, preference and other evidence lead to his using the drug at social events. A person might say that one should always tell the truth, but finds this difficult in situations where the truth might hurt someone, such as when giving a prognosis or commenting on appearance. Conflicts between patients and professionals, and between two professionals, can arise due to major ethical clashes (a health professional does not agree with termination but the patient is requesting this; a doctor agrees with euthanasia but a nurse does not) to issues that are more irritating than profound (I always finish a task staying on past 5pm at work if necessary, but my colleague is out the door 5 minutes before time to beat the car park rush). Volunteering or sticking up for one's values may be difficult in situations where there is a power differential. If your boss is always checking emails on his phone while you are talking to him, what can you do? But you would probably tell your 14 year old son not to do this.

Personal values are learnt through experience, through education and role modelling. As children we may at first assume our parents' and then our teachers' values. Later we are assaulted by a number of competing forces that may alter or reinforce our values. We learn what the consequences of our values-based choices are and decide to change these values. We mature.

If we change our behaviour in order to conform within the environment in which we work or live, but do not change our values we may become unhappy or burnout. For example, if we work within an office where it is acceptable for people to make sexist comments because no one challenges these, and everyone joins in, we may also laugh at the jokes while cringing inside. Eventually we either become acculturated to the behaviour or we continue to feel uneasy and feel discomfort at work. In the health care setting, profession X may make regular disparaging remarks about profession Y. As a member of X I do not initially join in, but neither do I stick up for Y, or challenge the remarks. I feel uncomfortable that I cannot uphold my values of fairness and equity, but am worried that I will be ostracised in the same way if I speak up. Members of Y probably think I am just like all the X's. Eventually I become a stereotypical X or have to move on. Similarly we may become immune to black humour and making fun of patients or health care situations. Older professionals may tell students that this is one way of dealing with stress and that, if kept within the profession, it will hurt no-one. But we do not work in professional silos, and we also work with non-professionals who make take great offence at this 'harmless fun'.

An important factor influencing learnt behaviour like this is the concept of what is called the 'hidden curriculum' (Hafferty & Franks, 1994) in relation to education, but which may be applied to any situation where learning from others may occur. In contrast to the intended or formal curriculum (what I intend learners to learn and which is explicit in terms of learning goals or outcomes), the hidden curriculum is learning by immersion, observation and role modelling. The hidden curriculum is 'the medium by which values and mores are transmitted, operates at many levels (from institutional down to an individual learning situation), and is without doubt one of the most powerful and unrealised influences on professional development' (Thistlethwaite & Spencer, 2008, page 166).

Communities, cultures and organisations may hold values in common. At some point these may have been discussed and agreed on by a majority of members. Later members are then assumed to agree with the values by virtue of their membership. An organisation may have a defined mission statement that all members learn about during induction; a community may have a code of conduct which if broken leads to punishment. However sometimes the communal values are not obvious until breached, and in defence an individual may state that she didn't know that what she did was wrong.

Professional values

Reflection point

What do you consider to be your profession's values? Do they differ from your personal values? Has anyone ever asked you what your professional values are? (Perhaps at interview?)

How do our professional values differ from our lifestyle and moral values? According to one management website (http://www.officearrow.com/job-satisfaction/what-are-your-professional-values-oaiur-636/view.html) professional values 'are the principles that guide your decisions and actions in your career'. We will consider later how values might differ between professions, but there is probably a core set with which all health and social care professionals would agree. This particular website calls these universal values, which should be held and practised within all professions. There are five (Box 1.3). Moreover, a failure to adhere to these values is believed to be a major cause of the economic and social damage that devastated the global economy in 2008.

Box 1.3: An example of professional values

- First, do no harm.
- Keep it simple.
- Honesty is the best policy.
- We're all in this together.
- Stay balanced.

The aphorism 'first, do no harm' is credited to Hippocrates, the father of medicine, and could be the motto of the patient safety movement. While this phrase was written in relation to not harming patients, we must also avoid harming our colleagues. We can harm both by commission and omission. To lessen the risk of harm health professionals learn to reflect-in-action: is what I am doing or planning to do likely to cause more harm than good? Sometimes in the heat of acute medical care there is little time to reflect, and little time to communicate, a potent cause of error.

Keep it simple: this may seem an impossible task in the modern complex world of patient care. The management angle on simplicity refers to transparency and openness. In health care this translates as professionals having an understanding of the roles and responsibilities of their colleagues: without this understanding should we be attempting to work together? If there is duplication of roles, we need to consider how best we might combine our efforts. When talking to each other while working, making referrals, discharging patients from one care-giver back to another, there should be clear language and explanations. There should rarely be the moment when one professional has to wonder: why he is doing that, why did she do that? If in doubt, ask. When asking a colleague to carry out a task, explain its purpose. Consider the possible advantages and disadvantages of each course of action, each step in the management plan. What are the possible benefits and risks? What risks are you, your colleagues and the patient prepared to take? Simplicity is also a key to good patient-professional communication: avoiding jargon and checking understanding.

Honesty is the best policy: being truthful is a commonly held value. Yet many of us use the 'little white lie' as a way out of difficult interactions. Being honest can be hurtful, and caring professionals are loathe to hurt and certainly to reduce hope. We say someone was brutally honest, suggesting that there are degrees of honesty. Consider the last time you were less than honest – would you translate this as actually lying? We say such things as: this won't hurt; there is nothing to worry about. If I don't list all the possible side effects of a medication, am I being honest? With colleagues we might say: you handled that quite well (but really we mean it could have been done better). Sometimes rather than be honest, we give feedback in different ways. If I am not happy with the way another health professional has dealt with *my* patient rather than tell them, I don't refer to that person again.

We're all in this together: can be read in many different ways. Perhaps it puts the onus on the professional to campaign for social justice and health equality. Perhaps it means we should think ecologically, about waste, about health costs. Or perhaps this reflects the values of professionalism that stress in times of difficulty we close ranks, we protect our own and we denigrate whistle-blowers. One of the six elements of a profession has been defined by a sociologist as organisation of members (Johnson, 1972). This organisation may also be regarded as professional autonomy and self-regulation, which some regard as a professional value:

'The central element of professional autonomy is the assurance that individual physicians have the freedom to exercise their professional judgment in the care and treatment of their patients…as a corollary to the right of professional autonomy, the medical profession has a continuing responsibility to be self-regulating…the medical profession itself must be responsible for regulating the professional conduct and activities of individual physicians' (The World Medical Association, 1987, online).

Values change and now in many countries such as the UK, the regulatory body includes lay representatives who judge professional conduct.

Balance: as health professionals we should role model good health practices, including the work-life balance. We teach self-care to health professional students, and then wonder why they do not want to work long hours, or stay late to ensure their patients have some continuity of care. But for our own well-being we do need to balance our clients' needs and our own. We also need to balance our colleagues' needs, the team's needs and our family's.

Examples of professional values

What are the similarities and differences in values between health care professions? We can explore these in part by looking at the documentation of health professions containing their stated values or principles of good practice.

For doctors in the UK the General Medical Council has a number of publications focusing on good medical practice. These include the duties of a doctor, which incorporate values

(Box 1.4). The GMC also now states that doctors must inform the council if they believe a colleague is unfit to practise. This 'telling tales' may go against some doctors' values.

Box 1.4: Duties of a doctor – selected examples (General Medical Council, 2002)

- Make the care of the patient your first concern.
- Treat every patient politely and considerately.
- Respect patients' dignity and privacy.
- Listen to patients and respect their views
- Respect the rights of patients to be fully involved in decisions about their care.
- Be honest and trustworthy.
- Respect and protect confidential information.
- Make sure that your personal beliefs do not prejudice your patients' care.
- Avoid abusing your position as a doctor.
- Work with colleagues in the ways that best serve patients' interests.

In one study nurses have identified human dignity, equality among patients and prevention of suffering as their top ranking professional values (Rassin, 2008). These resonate with the Australian Code of Ethics for Nurses, which lists eight items that nurses value (Box 1.5). There are obvious overlaps between nursing and medicine. The allied health professions have similar statements but there is not enough room to list all of these.

Box 1.5: Code of ethics for nurses (Australian Nursing and Midwifery Council, 2008)

Nurses value:

- Quality nursing care for patients.
- Respect and kindness for self and others.
- The diversity of people.
- Access for quality nursing and health care for all people.
- Informed decision making.
- Cultures of safety in nursing and health care.
- Ethical management of information.
- A socially, economically and ecologically sustainable environment promoting health and well-being.

The 10 principles of values-based practice

There are 10 principles of VBP under four headings (Box 1.6). I will consider the implications of these in the context of interprofessional teamwork.

Health professionals need to be aware of the values in a given situation; this also means not assuming what someone's values might be. When in doubt, ask. It is easy to make a value judgment about other people, and other professionals, leading to miscommunication which may not be apparent straight away but which may ultimately cause difficulty with sharing care and decisions. Reasoning then is about thinking of these values when making decisions. We need to know about values and facts that are relevant to a situation, and have some knowledge about how the professions might differ in their professional values as members of multidisciplinary or interprofessional teams. Good communication helps resolve conflicts.

Box 1.6: The 10 principles of values-based practice (Fulford, 2004; Woodbridge and Fulford, 2004, page 20)

Practice skills

1. Awareness: of the values present in a given situation.
2. Reasoning: using a clear reasoning process to explore the values present when making decisions.
3. Knowledge: of the values and facts relevant to the specific situation.
4. Communication: combined with the previous three skills is central to the resolution of conflicts and the decision making process.

Models of service delivery

5. User-centred: the first source for information on values is the perspective of the service user.
6. Multidisciplinary: as in teamworking (see also interprofessional).

VBP and Evidence-based practice (EBP)

7. The two-feet principle: all decisions are based on facts and values.
8. The 'squeaky wheel' principle: we only notice values when there is a problem.
9. Science and values: increasing scientific knowledge creates choices in health care, and therefore wide differences in values.
10. Partnership: decisions are taken by service users and providers of care in partnership.

The 'two feet' principle is that all decisions are based on facts and values. Evidence-based practice and values-based practice are complementary and both need to be considered. Can you think of instances where professionals use different evidence bases because of their different literatures and research approaches? The 'squeaky wheel' principle is that values shouldn't just be noticed if there's a problem.

Increasing scientific knowledge creates choices in health care. This can lead to wider differences in values. Shared decision making is important when there is choice – shared between patient and professional, and between the different professionals involved in partnership. This may not be as easy or uncontroversial as it sounds. In particular the professionals may not work in partnership together for a number of reasons, which we explore in this book.

Patient-centred practice

VBP should be a fundamental part of patient-centred care, and indeed the two approaches may be considered to be very similar. A major difference is that patient-centred care 'centres on the patient', encompassing an exploration of the patient's values but not specifically the professional's.

At this point, it is worth considering the meaning of patient centredness, a term that is not easily defined. The patient-centred approach to patient-professional interaction is based on the premise that a patient's problem may be defined in terms of its physical, psychological and social components, what has been called the biopsychosocial model (Engel 1960; 1980); more recently some practitioners are also adding the dimension of spirituality. Nearly 30 years ago in the classic text about general practice consultations, the recommendation to explore a patient's ideas, concerns and expectations became linked to patient centredness; thus: '…it would seem that satisfaction of the patient is more likely when the doctor discovers and deals with the patient's concerns and expectations; when the doctor's manner communicates warmth, interest and concern about the patients, when the doctor volunteers a lot of information and explains things to the patient in terms that are understood' (Pendleton, 1983, page 45). To these three elements we are now adding values, but with the extra emphasis on sharing of values, in a two-way reciprocal process.

The easiest way to define patient-centredness relies on tautology: it involves putting the patient at the centre or focus of the interaction. In the next chapter on teamwork, we will also find that we are exhorted to put the patient at the centre of the team. Yet, if we are aiming to build a partnership, 'a meeting between experts', and the patient is in the centre, where is the professional?

The expert patient

The idea of the patient as an expert was put forward in the 1985 book *Meeting between experts* (Tuckett et al., 1985) and focused on shared understanding between patient and practitioner. The patient was defined as an expert about his or her illness. The doctor, in this case, would ask about a patient's ideas about the illness or problem, he or she would then tap into this expertise and share his or her own professional diagnosis of the problem in turn with the patient. The result should be shared understanding, with both parties being aware of any points of conflict and differences between each other. Of course we now know that some of this conflict arises from disparate values, which are not specifically mentioned.

Communication skills training is now a major part of health professional curricula. Practitioners learn how to be patient (or client) centred. However, many patients remain unused to interacting in such a way. They, of course, receive no formal training in such interactions: they learn on the job, in the consultation, from the cues they are given about what may or may not be discussed. Many patients also worry about wasting a doctor's time with problems they perceive as non-medical (Bensing, 1991). When asked to share ideas, concerns and values, patients may find it difficult to express these, and their feelings, particularly if they do not do this regularly. Skilled professionals should be more able to put patients at their ease and facilitate two-way communication. But even these practitioners may not be used to considering how their own values impact on the care they deliver.

Barriers to VBP

As good communication is a necessity for VBP, the barriers to VBP are also the factors that impede communication. These factors can be thought of under three headings (Thistlethwaite & Morris, 2006).

Professional/practitioner factors

The predominant barrier is lack of training and lack of awareness of the different approaches to improving communication. Professionals may also focus on the tasks of the consultation/interaction such as health promotion and diagnosis, and neglect the process such as establishing rapport and involving patients in decisions. Some practitioners are reluctant to explore patient concerns because of worries about feeling powerless or overwhelmed by patients' problems. This feeling may be heightened if the professional has trouble dealing with uncertainty, lacks empathy and/or feels burnt out.

Patient factors

Patients, on the whole, need to be invited to discuss their concerns and values. They are usually reticent in volunteering information when the professional is eliciting a formal medical history. As noted above they may be concerned about wasting the practitioner's time. Their values may be very personal and not something they have much practice in discussing. They may be embarrassed to divulge values, particularly if they consider them likely to be at odds with those of the person they are consulting.

Organisational factors

The main barrier is time. Consultations in general practice tend to be fairly short: up to 10 minutes with a GP, maybe 20 minutes with a practice nurse, possibly more with other health professionals for treatment, e.g., physiotherapy, counselling, social work. Professionals often feel frustration with lack of resources; inviting patients to discuss concerns and share decisions, taking into account ideas and values, result in a management choice that is not feasible within the local health service.

Evidence-based practice

VBP complements evidence-based practice, though the latter is usually referred to as evidence-based medicine (EBM), reflecting the biomedical positivist culture, with its emphasis that all clinical decisions and management plans should have supporting evidence.

A useful definition of evidence-based medicine (EBM) is:

'... the conscientious, explicit, and judicious use of current best evidence in making decisions about the care of individual patients. The practice of evidence based medicine means integrating individual clinical expertise with the best available external clinical evidence from systematic research. By individual clinical expertise we mean the proficiency and judgment that individual clinicians acquire through clinical experience and clinical practice. Increased expertise is reflected in many ways, but especially in more effective and efficient diagnosis and in the more thoughtful identification and compassionate use of individual patients' predicaments, rights, and preferences in making clinical decisions about their care. By best available external clinical evidence we mean clinically relevant research, often from the basic sciences of medicine, but especially from patient centred clinical research into the accuracy and precision of diagnostic tests (including the clinical examination), the power of prognostic markers, and the efficacy and safety of therapeutic, rehabilitative, and preventive regimens. External clinical evidence both invalidates previously accepted diagnostic tests and treatments and replaces them with new ones that are more powerful, more accurate, more efficacious, and safer'.

(Sackett et al., 1996)

Note the reference to patients' predicaments, rights and preferences rather than values.

Thus, according to the EBM movement, all investigations and treatment should be evidence based. Problems arise when there is no evidence, it is conflicting or potentially out-of-date. The evidence may also recommend management that is not available in the local health service, is considered too expensive and unlikely to be funded, or is outside the professional's area of expertise. The 'best' option may not always be what the patient would choose, but this raises the question as to who defines 'best'.

Health professionals are expected to keep up-to-date with advances in medical knowledge and published evidence. But the speed with which the discipline is changing makes it almost impossible for generalists, such as work in primary care, to be abreast of all recent developments. Clinicians are often confronted by clinical questions and patient expectations that cannot be answered or met on the spot. There is a greater reliance on technology to provide quick answers to dilemmas, to help clinicians search for evidence. They also need to be able to evaluate such information and evidence, plus the information that patients provide, which they may have gleaned from the media and Internet. Working through the evidence with the patient, taking into account that individual's preferences, is challenging work.

Putting the results of research evidence into practice is known as knowledge translation: the exchange, synthesis and ethically sound application of knowledge, within a complex system of interactions among researchers and users, to accelerate the capture of the benefits of research (CIHR, 2004).

However, clinicians' interpretation and use of research findings will always be based on their experience and values. They need to be aware of this and how it not only influences their decision-making but the information they share with patients. A problem with clinical trials is that the participants in such trials are usually very different to the patient in your own clinical interaction. Professionals work very much within a 'trial of one' framework: if you prescribe or recommend a particular treatment, which has adverse effects for that patient, you are less likely to adopt that approach again. This trial of one method is consistent with the theory that doctors make diagnostic and treatment decisions based on the 'illness scripts' of their previous patients (Schmidt et al., 1990).

The increasing number of evidence-based guidelines, protocols and frameworks are affecting professional and patient autonomy in respect of decision-making. Some practitioners are concerned that if they do not follow recommendations, they could face professional reprobation or legal challenges from families. Working through what is often confusing and difficult wording to help patients make decisions about risk and benefits is time consuming, and it is difficult to be sure that the patients and/or carer has really understood the options and the potential outcomes. There are tools to help with this process, including decision aids both paper-based and online.

Of interest in relation to EBM is a book by Freshwater and Rolfe (2004), which deconstructs the concept in the style of the French philosopher Derrida. They state that the paper that introduced EBM to the world (Evidence-based Medicine Working Group, 1992) was 'full of ambiguity, evasion and contradiction' (page 83) and justify these comments at length. This highlights how individuals and professionals interpret, use and value 'evidence' in different ways.

Conclusion

There are a number of definitions of values and values-based practice. There are also published lists of values relating to particular professions, which may or may not resonate with an individual's personal values. Sharing values as team members is important and in the next chapter we consider teamwork in more detail from this perspective.

References

Allport GW. (1961). *Pattern and growth in personality*. New York: Holt, Rinehart and Winston. p454.

Australian Government: Australian Department of Immigration and Citizenship. (2011). Available at: www.immi.gov.au/

living-in-australia/values/statement/long/ (Accessed December 2011).

Australian Nursing and Midwifery Council. (2008). *Code of ethics for nurses in Australia*. Available at: www.nrgpn.org.au/index. php?element=ANMC±Code±of±Ethics (Accessed December 2011).

Bensing J. (1991). Doctor-patient communication and the quality of care. *Social Science and Medicine*, **32**; 1301–1310.

CIHR. (2004). *Knowledge translation strategy 2004–2009: innovation in action*. Ottawa, ON: Canadian Institutes of Health Research.

Engel GL. (1960). A unified concept of health and disease. *Perspectives in Biology and Medicine*, 3;459–485.

Engel GL. (1980). The clinical application of the biopsychosocial model. *American Journal of Psychiatry*, **137**;535–543.

Evidence-Based Medicine Working Group. (1992). Evidence-based medicine: a new approach to teaching the practice of medicine. *Journal of the American Medical Association*, **268**;2420–2425.

Freshwater D and Rolfe G. (2004). *Deconstructing evidence-based practice*. Abingdon: Routledge.

Fulford KWM. (2004). Ten principles of values-based medicine. In: Radden J. (Ed). *The philosophy of psychiatry: a companion*. New York: Oxford University Press. p205–234.

Fulford KWM, Peile E and Carroll H. (2012). *Essential values-based practice*. Cambridge: Cambridge University Press.

General Medical Council. (2002). *The duties of a doctor*. London: GMC.

Hafferty FW and Franks R. (1994). The hidden curriculum, ethics teaching and the structure of medical education. *Academic Medicine*, **30**;861–871.

Johnson TJ. (1972). *Professions and power*. London: Macmillan Press Limited.

Mason T, Hinman P, Sadik R, Collyer D, Hosker N and Keen A. (2010). Values of reductionism and values of holism. In: McCarthy J & Rose P (Eds). *Values-based health and social care. Beyond evidence-based practice*. London: Sage. p70–96.

National Institute for Mental Health in England. Available at: www.nmhdu.org.uk/our-work/ improving-mental-health-care-pathways/ implementing-the-amended-mental-health-act-1983/training/value-based-practice/ ?keywords=values (Accessed December 2011).

Pendleton D. (1983). Doctor-patient communication: a review. In: Pendleton D & Hasler J (Eds). *Doctor-patient communication*. London: Academic Press, p5–56.

Rassin M. (2008). Nurses' professional and personal values. *Nursing Ethics*, **15**; 614–630.

Royal College of General Practitioners. (2007). *Clinical ethics and values-based practice*. Available at: www.rcgp-curriculum.org.uk/ pdf/curr_3_3_Clinical_ethics.pdf (Accessed December 2011).

Sackett DL, Rosenberg WMC, Muir Gray JA, Haynes RB and Richardson WS. (1996). Evidence-based medicine: what it is and what it isn't. *BMJ*, **312**;71–72.

Schmidt HG, Norman GR and Boshuizen HPA. (1990). A cognitive perspective on medical expertise: theory and implications. *Academic Medicine*, **65**;611–621.

Seedhouse D. (2005). *Values-based decision making for the caring professions*. Chichester: John Wiley & Sons.

Thistlethwaite JE and Morris P. (2006). *Patient-doctor consultations in primary care: theory and practice*. London: RCGP.

Thistlethwaite JE and Spencer J. (2008). *Professionalism in medicine*. Oxford: Radcliffe Medical Press.

Thomas M, Burt M and Parkes J. (2010). The emergence of evidence-based practice. In: McCarthy J & Rose P (Eds). *Values-based health and social care. Beyond evidence-based practice*. London: Sage. p3–24.

Thornton T. (2006). Tacit knowledge as the unifying factor in evidence based medicine and clinical judgement. *Philosophy, Ethics, and Humanities in Medicine*, 1;E2.

Tuckett D, Boulton M, Olson C and Williams A. (1985). *Meetings between experts. An approach to sharing ideas in medical consultations*. London: Tavistock Publications.

University of Lincoln. Available at: http://www.lincoln.ac.uk/ccawi/esc/New_Folder/module-4.pdf (Accessed December 2011).

Warne T and McAndrew S. (2008). Value. In: Whitehead-Mason E, McIntosh A, Bryan A & Mason t (Eds). *Key concepts in nursing.* London: Sage. p315–321.

Woodbridge K and Fulford KWM. (2004). *Whose values? A workbook for values-based practice in mental health care.* London: The Sainsbury Centre for Mental Health.

World Medical Association. Available at: www.wma.net/e/policy/a21.htm (Accessed December 2011).

Chapter

2

Teamwork and collaborative practice in modern health care

This chapter explores the concept and practice of teamwork and collaboration in health care delivery, including the importance of professionalism, professional identity and training. We consider how goals and values may vary according to one's profession, training and experiences, and team membership.

Modern twenty-first century health care delivery within developed countries is complex, often highly specialised and most commonly carried out by teams of health professionals. The professional workforce is diverse and the professions within it have many different roles and responsibilities. Their professional language also differs to some extent, the most notable example being in relation to the recipient of their care with nomenclature including patient, client, service user and even consumer. A patient, or client, is unlikely to interact with only one type of professional during what is now commonly referred to as the 'patient journey', i.e. a person's experience of and movement through the health care system during the course of an illness or condition. Patients with chronic diseases, such as diabetes, ischaemic heart disease and mental health problems, will consult with many different health and social care professionals, be referred between services and locations, and have to discuss their ideas and management many times. In 1999 a British study showed that patients with cancer interacted with 28 doctors during the first year after diagnosis (Smith et al. 1999), not counting the other health professionals involved in both primary and secondary care.

While many of these clinicians will work in well-defined teams, some will only have loose affiliations with other staff, raising questions of definitions of teamwork and leadership. Moreover patients may choose to consult practitioners outside the health service, and to access complementary and alternative therapists (CAM), as well as the doctors, nurses, physiotherapists, psychologists etc who are considered part of mainstream care delivery. It is rare that many of these people will be co-located, that they will meet regularly, if at all, that they will share common values and that they will be able to communicate in a timely and constructive manner. Patients, thus, are likely to receive conflicting messages, enhancing the chances of misunderstandings, and are often unsure of who has overall responsibility for their treatment and care. How can this situation be improved and what role does values-based practice have in teamwork and collaboration? The particular issues with communication will be dealt with in chapter 3; this chapter will focus on other aspects of teamwork.

The health care team

Many health and social care professionals are not grouped together in 'official' teams during their interacting with the same patients, families and carers. Moreover many of these commonly work within strict boundaries set by their professional bodies and this can be frustrating for some who prefer a greater flexibility in patient care. Professions have hierarchical lines of authority and different levels of professional autonomy. A nurse may be in a health care team but be line managed by someone other than the team leaders, another nurse higher up in the professional hierarchy; similarly with allied health professionals.

What is teamwork?

Over a decade ago, the Institute of Medicine in the USA recognised effective teamwork as a means of coping with the increasing complexity and technological advances in diagnosis and health care delivery (Institute of Medicine, 2001). There is a large body of literature relating to teamwork in health and other complex organisations, sport and education. We can learn from other disciplines while keeping sight of potential differences in health and social care, particularly if we take into consideration the emphasis on the patient (or client) or family-centred approach to delivery, and its corollary: the patient at the centre of the team.

Definitions of a team

There are many definitions of a team and teamwork but there are common themes within them (Box 2.1).

Box 2.1: Definitions of a team

'A team is a small number of people with complementary skills, who are committed to a common purpose, performance, goals and approach, for which they are mutually accountable.
High performance team members are … committed to one another.'
(Hammick et al., 2009, page 39)
'Teamwork is the way people work together cooperatively and effectively.'
(Manion et al., 1996, page 4)
'A group may be defined as a number of individuals who join together to achieve a goal' whereas *'a team is a set of interpersonal relationships structured to achieve established goals'*. (Johnson & Johnson, 2006 page 5, page 595)
Katzenbach and Smith (1993) include values in their definition:
'Teamwork represents a set of values that encourage behaviours such as listening and constructively responding to points of view expressed by others, giving others the benefit of the doubt, providing support to those who need it, and recognising the interests and achievements of others'
(page 15).

Researchers at Aston University in the UK have described three conditions necessary for functioning teamwork (Dawson et al., 2007); they talk of objectives rather than goals:

- Clear objectives that are known to all members.
- Team members work closely together to achieve these objectives.
- There are regular meetings to review team effectiveness and discuss how it can be improved.

These conditions do not include a discussion about team or individual values, though discussions about team effectiveness may encompass values if there are problems relating to diversity that need to be improved.

Common themes/words from teamwork definitions are: size, communication, working together, review, responsibility and respect. The optimum size for a team is not mentioned, but the business literature suggests that it is between 5 and 10. If we think of core and wider health care teams, numbers may be much larger than this. Taking the different perspectives and definitions into account there appears to be a common set of requirements for generic team working (Box 2.2). Are shared values imperative and is this possible? We may have to compromise and state: awareness of shared and diverse values and the affect of these.

Box 2.2: Requirements for effective teams (from Reeves et al., 2010)

- Clear team goals.
- Shared team commitment.
- Role clarity.
- Interdependence.
- Integration between team members.

For health care teams, and in particular teams with a diverse professional membership, a number of other features have been suggested as being important (Box 2.3). As Reeves et al. (2010) point out this list is largely theoretical and inspirational without conclusive empirical evidence as to how the factors affect quality team working in practice. Here the mention of values is related to valuing and respecting each other rather than focusing on the values of team members, though 'democratic approaches' could be seen as a team value in itself.

The list in Box 2.3 focuses on co-located teams, i.e. health professionals working in one health centre or clinic, or perhaps in one geographical area but with a common meeting place (e.g. some professionals based in the clinic, some in the wider community, but with offices in the same building thus facilitating regular formal and informal meetings). In health care however we can also think of a much wider team of professionals including social workers

> **Box 2.3:** Attributes of functional health care teams: from Reeves et al. (2010), drawing on the work of West and Slater (1996) with primary care teams, and Hammick et al. (2009)
>
> - Democratic approaches.
> - Agreeing ground rules and processes for working together.
> - An understanding of values, knowledge and skills of team members.
> - Active participation by all members.
> - Efforts to breakdown stereotypes and barriers.
> - Regular time to develop team working away from practice.
> - Good communication.
> - A single shared work location.
> - Mutual role understanding.
> - The development of joint protocols, training and work practices.
> - Agreed practice priorities across professional boundaries.
> - Regular and effective team meetings.
> - Team members valuing and respecting each other.
> - Maintaining professional relationships.
> - Good performance management.

and secondary care practitioners, and even in some cases teachers, psychologists and probation officers. This is a different type of team working as the membership is fluid, the meetings rare, the hierarchies and lines of reporting different and the likelihood of shared goal setting rare. The further away a professional is from the central team, the less likely it is that he or she will be able to discuss or share values, and the more likely it is that roles may be misunderstood and patient care fragmented.

Team membership: homogeneity and heterogeneity

During our lives we work in and know of many teams. In secondary and higher education there is often team-based learning. In our early teams, while there may be differences between members such as gender and ethnicity, there were likely to be many similarities: age, studying the same subjects and sitting the same examinations, aiming for the same profession, perhaps (at some schools) having the same religion, etc. In some situations team members would also have similar values. In our working lives, teams are likely to be much more heterogeneous: different ages, professions, experiences, knowledge and skills, responsibilities (personal and work-related).

One theory of team development is discussed frequently, though there is a lack of empirical data as to its validity across different types of teams (Box 2.4). The theory relates to new teams rather than a new member joining an existing team. In the clinical environment a completely new team may be convened to offer new services, or if, for example, a new health centre is opened. But in the main team membership changes over time as well-established teams evolve.

Interprofessional and multiprofessional team work

Adjectives highlighting the diversity of membership applied to teamwork within the health sphere are: multiprofessional, interprofessional, multidisciplinary and others. While these words are often used interchangeably and without formal definitions, there is a growing consensus as to the meaning of some and their prefixes.

Box 2.4: Stages of team development (from Tuckman & Jensen 1977)

- Forming – everyone tends to be nice to each other, sounding each other out, should define and agree team goals and values.
- Storming – questioning of goals and values, particularly each other's values as people become more relaxed and outspoken and no longer concentrate on masking attitudes; can be useful to bring buried tensions out into the open.
- Norming – normality is resumed, communication is better: members listen to each other and there is mutual respect.
- Performing – effective and productive work, begins to meet goals.
- Adjourning – project-based teams have a natural end point (unlike many health care teams).

As *inter* means between, among and mutually, the interprofessional approach to patient care may be defined as involving practitioners from different professional backgrounds delivering services and coordinating care programmes to achieve different and often disparate service client needs. Ideally goals are set collaboratively (including with the patient) through consensual decision-making. The result should be an individualised patient care plan, which may be delivered by one or more professionals. This level of collaborative practice is difficult to achieve but does maximise the value of shared expertise. (This definition draws on work from a number of sources and is listed in a glossary compiled by the WHO's study group on interprofessional education and collaborative practice in 2010.)

Multi, with its connotations of many, leads to a definition of multiprofessional as: two or more professionals working side by side, without any particular cooperation or collaboration.

Interprofessional teamworking

In the UK, there have been a number of national reports on health system renewal from an interprofessional perspective published. The Department of Health in 2004 funded 'Creating an Interprofessional Workforce: an education and training framework for health and social care in England (CIPW)', based on the premise that 'effective leadership, teamwork and management support are the bedrock of collaboration in health and social care' (Department of Health, 2007). Highlighting again the issues with terminology, the Department for Education and Skills published *Every Child Matters* in the same year, which advocated *multi-disciplinary* teams and the enhancement of relationships between health and social care professionals, the police and teachers (Department for Education and Skills, 2004).

Team functioning

Optimum team functioning, as mentioned above, seems to be dependent on common goal settings, regular meetings and reflection on performance. Health professionals who have identified themselves as working in teams but who did not meet all three of these parameters have reported less job satisfaction and more burnout, with a greater likelihood of patient safety issues (Dawson et al., 2007).

How does one gain an understanding of the values, knowledge and skills of team members, and the overarching values of the team collectively? Orientation within new teams and new working environments is important. Some of the knowledge will be gained through working together, but this cannot be assumed. How often is there a reiteration of the team's values and working practices when a new member joins? How often is the new member encouraged to discuss his or her own values, as well as the knowledge and skills brought to the team? Everyone has pre-existing ideas about and expectations of their new colleagues and workplace. Some of these may be based on previous experience, some on the stories of previous colleagues, some on media reports and pre-reading. It is important that a new team member is aware of any biases or prejudices arising from stereotyping, their own professional culture, their gender or their age.

Dysfunctional teams

There are a number of types of dysfunctional teams, some more common in health care than others (Field, 2009). The team may be working as a group of individuals: the value here is everyone for him or herself (which raises the question as to whether this is a team at all). As health professionals there may still be a commitment to the patient, but the individual makes sure that he or she does not work the longest hours, or see the most patients. The GP may rarely ask for someone else's opinion; this doctor is not used to working in a team. Factional teams are more likely in that individual team members identify more with their profession and their own professional colleagues than with the multiprofessional team members. The professions seek each other out and sit together when possible. Some teams avoid conflict, yet working through conflict rather than burying and ignoring it can make a team stronger and more productive. Then there is the indecisive team. There are so many areas to work on but prioritisation is difficult: what shall we do about improving our care to patients with asthma? Should we focus on asthma rather than diabetes? But Mary thinks the main problem is depression and we aren't diagnosing that enough.

Not all dysfunctional teams are alike but five common characteristics of dysfunctional teams have been identified (Box 2.5). The first, emphasising the need for trust, highlights the vulnerability of some team members. Trust may be a defined core value of the team: we need to trust each other to be able to work together. Trust is lost for many reasons. Sometimes an individual health professional has lost trust in a whole other professional group because of bad experiences. 'I cannot trust the nurses to do that, I'd better do it myself.' This lack of trust may also be related to not fully understanding the role of other health professionals, what they have been trained to do and are competent at: if in doubt, the best thing is to ask. Building and maintaining trust requires regular interactions and discussion of near misses and significant events.

Box 2.5: Five characteristics of dysfunctional teams (Lencioni, 2002)

- Absence of trust.
- Fear of conflict.
- Lack of commitment.
- Avoidance of accountability.
- Inattention to results.

We have already discussed the need to agree on goals. But what if one team member is not committed to those goals? Strictly speaking if someone was opposed to a particular goal, it should not have been included without debate and consensus. But once a team is dysfunctioning, it is hard to admit to lack of commitment and so the goal is undermined more subtly. One professional may tell a patient: I don't agree with that medication, or that dose. Or 'why did the nurse do that to you?'

Dealing with such issues is going to mean conflict, but dysfunctional teams often avoid conflict, and therefore do not air their differences so they can be openly discussed. Conflict does not mean a full slanging match with insult trading. Conflict can be productive if there are ground rules and respect so each voice is heard. If there is conflict about a particular issue, once this seems to have been resolved, ensure that each team member is committed to the outcome and is not going to undermine the consensus view.

Dysfunctional teams may be helped by team meetings, sometimes with outside consultants, to help build team morale and diagnose difficulties. There needs to be a certain amount of self-awareness to note that the team is not functioning and needs help. Often the leadership is a problem, and the leader may be blind to this, causing a reluctance to seek assistance.

Reflection point

Think about your teams past and present. Did/do they function well? How do you measure functionality? Have you worked in a dysfunctioning team? Reflect on the effect this had on you, your colleagues and your patients/clients. How did you resolve the problem?

Collaboration: what's in a name?

I have mentioned the word collaboration a number of times above. Indeed the literature on teamwork is increasingly concerned with collaboration, an interesting word as one of its dictionary definitions highlights its meaning of 'working with the enemy'. Collaboration is also used in its adverbial form to describe a function of teamwork: teams are often defined by their actions: one such action is working collaboratively together. Collaborative practice is a newer term in this context: is collaborative practice synonymous with teamwork?

Reflection point

What do you understand by collaboration? Does it differ from teamwork? What makes a good collaborator?

Reeves et al. (2010) have conceptualised the relationships between these terms as a series of widening circles (Figure 2.1). In the centre circle is interprofessional teamwork as "the most 'focused' of activities with high levels of interdependence, integration and shared responsibility" (p44). From here we ripple out to collaboration, coordination and networking. Thus collaboration means working together but with reduced levels of interdependence, integration and shared responsibility. Your number of collaborators is likely to be much higher than 10.

Reflection point

Considering the different forms of interprofessional work, where would you put the professionals with whom you interact and provide patient care? Who are your immediate team?

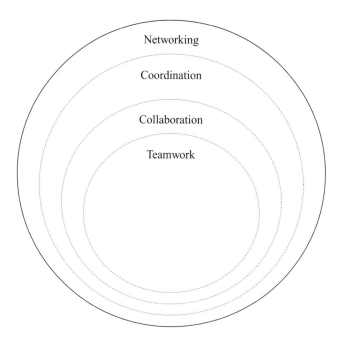

Figure 2.1. Differing forms of interprofessional work (Reeves et al., 2010, page 44). Reproduced with permission from Wiley-Blackwell.

Collaborative practice

Collaborative practice is a priority of the World Health Organization (WHO), which published its *Framework for Action on Interprofessional Action and Collaborative Practice* in 2010. Definitions of collaborative practice are given in Box 2.6.

Box 2.6: Definitions of collaborative practice

'A collaborative practice-ready health worker is someone who has learned how to work in an interprofessional team and is competent to do so.

Collaborative practice happens when multiple health workers from different professional backgrounds work together with patients, families, carers and communities to deliver the highest quality of care. It allows health workers to engage any individual whose skills can help achieve local health goals.'

'Interprofessional collaboration is the process of developing and maintaining effective interprofessional working relationships with learners, practitioners, patients/clients/ families and communities to enable optimal health outcomes. Elements of collaboration include respect, trust, shared decision making, and partnerships.'

Canadian Interprofessional Health Collaborative (CIHC).

The CIHC goes onto state:

'For interprofessional teams of learners and practitioners to work collaboratively, the integration of role clarification, team functioning, collaborative leadership, and a patient/client/family/community-centred focus to care/services is supported through interprofessional communication. Effective interprofessional communication is dependent on the ability of teams to deal with conflicting viewpoints and reach reasonable compromises.'

The business organisational literature has interesting and different discussions about the meaning of collaboration. In 2007 academics from Indiana University, writing in the Journal of Public Administration Research and Theory, declared that 'collaboration is emerging as a distinct focus of scholarly research' and that while the literature is multidisciplinary and extensive 'it also lacks coherence across disciplines' (Thomson et al., 2009, page 23). Moreover there are many definitions of collaboration across the different literatures. Thomson et al. (2009), through a review of published work and interviews, formulate the following definition:

'Collaboration is a process in which autonomous or semi-autonomous actors interact through formal and informal negotiation, jointly creating rules and structures governing their relationships and ways to act or decide on the issues that brought them together; it is a process involving shared norms and mutually beneficial interactions' (page 25).

Interesting words here are autonomous/semi-autonomous; formal/informal and shared norms. The concept of autonomy within health care practice is often used to refer to being able to work without supervision, but it is also referred to a requirement of being a professional: 'professional autonomy'. Norms are the rules of behaviour arising from the ideology of the team members, which reflect their values. Such behaviour is therefore either right and proper, or inappropriate. In this definition norms are the behaviours arising from the attitudes including values.

The authors of the above definition of collaboration emphasise that it is a multidimensional construct composed of five key dimensions: governance, administration, mutuality, norms and organisational autonomy. If we consider each of these with reference to health care delivery we can begin to understand the complexity of the process. In terms of governance, health professionals need to be able to make decisions together as to how they will work and behave, and what sort of relationships they will have. This could be seen as setting ground rules for working together, but there needs to be flexibility depending on the patient/client interaction and the patient/client needs.

A collaboration of health professionals, which is not a highly defined team, needs to be administered, or project managed, to ensure good communication and task processing. The administrator or manager, who is not necessarily the leader, arranges meetings, ensures information is passed between the professionals and the patients, and organises the timeline for action.

Mutuality is based around shared interests; in health care this focuses on the interests of the patient, but such interests need to be defined, explored and shared. Sharing and consensus may not come naturally, and may involve conflict and negotiation, the conflict arising sometimes due to conflicting values and lack of communication.

Norms, as mentioned above, resonate with values. Organisational autonomy is important in health care. Health professionals maintain their professional and individual identities while having to take on collaborative identities with their co-workers. Professional values and personal values may conflict, as professional autonomy creates a tension with the collective interest. Good collaborative practice therefore, like teamwork, requires skills of negotiation, conflict resolution and compromise. The WHO states that there is now evidence to show that collaborative practice enhances health services and improves health outcomes, particularly for patients with chronic diseases (WHO, 2010). Collaborative practice also appears to improve patient safety, reduce the length of hospital stay and the number of admissions, increase patient and carer satisfaction and promotes adherence to treatment plans.

Another way of conceptualising the way in which health care professionals interact is the notion of relational coordination. This term is the focus of a book on *High Performance Healthcare* by an American professor of management (Gittell, 2009). The thesis of her work is that there is commonly a lack of coordination between health professionals working in hospitals and, based on research in health care organisations, she describes how organisations delivering health care could 'harness the power of relationships to achieve and sustain high performance over time…' (page xiii). High performance is measured by patient outcomes including satisfaction, length of hospital stay and safety, as well as staff satisfaction and motivation. Relational coordination is defined as 'coordinating work through relationships of shared goals, shared knowledge and mutual respect'. These obviously overlap with the Aston imperatives and, while there is no explicit mention of values, these would surely underlie the setting of shared goals and the mutual respect generated and necessary.

Competencies for team work and interprofessional collaborative practice

Reflection point

What does an individual need to know and be able to do in order to be an effective team member? Can team work be learnt? Are team working skills generic or are they context specific, i.e. dependent on the membership of the team, the size of the team, the working environment and the leadership?

Educators within the health care field have been working during the last decades on developing a set of competencies required for optimal collaborative practice. One definition of competency includes values in terms of being the integrated application of not only knowledge and skills, but also values, experience, contacts, external knowledge resources and tools to solve a problem or to perform an activity (Kunzmann, 2006).

The Canadian Interprofessional Health Collaborative (CIHC) has produced a national interprofessional competency framework (2010), which refers to values in its document:

'Six competency domains highlight the knowledge, skills, attitudes and values that shape the judgments essential for interprofessional collaborative practice'.

The competency domains are listed in Box 2.7. Each of these domains is further described and explained. Under team functioning the necessary requirements include that practitioners are able to 'develop a set of principles for working together that respect the ethical values of members'. Under team ethics are the following items: confidentiality, resource allocation and professionalism.

Box 2.7: Competencies for interprofessional practice

- Interprofessional communication.
- Patient/client/family/community-centred care.
- Role clarification.
- Team functioning.
- Collaborative leadership.
- Interprofessional conflict resolution.

Reflection point

Consider you own working environment. Given what you have read, would you define yourself as working in a team? If so, think who are the members of this team. Do you meet regularly to set and review your goals? Perhaps you feel that the ultimate goal is better patient care and that you do not need to break this goal down into smaller chunks. Is this goal your team's value? Has your team ever discussed this goal explicitly and thought how best to achieve it? Have you, indeed, ever stopped to define what better patient care is? Do you feel that a health care professional is the best person to define care?

Maybe you think that you should involve patients in defining their goals for care. Patients often have different goals from our own. The British quality outcomes framework (QoF) for general practice sets targets (goals) for primary care teams which can be measured against objective standards, for example blood glucose control, blood pressure. The language involved is interesting. The value of a blood sugar is measured in millimoles per litre, and a blood pressure in millimetres of mercury. While some patients like to know, record and check that their values are within normal range, this type of value is very different to those of VBP. What sorts of goals does your team and your wider collaborative value? How might your patients judge the performance of your team?

The last question above is important. Sharon Mickan, from Australia, has researched into the characteristics of effective teams and found that 'team members and stakeholders commonly judge and prioritise effect team performance differently' (Mickan, 2005, page 215).

Professional stereotypes: a barrier to collaborative practice

Think of the first words that come into your head when someone says: doctor, specialist, general practitioner, nurse, midwife, matron, physiotherapist, orthopaedic surgeon, psychologist, pharmacist, ward clerk, receptionist. Chances are that you think of stereotypical images of these roles, affected somewhat by your own profession and your experience. The images are steeped in your own values and those you relate to the job in question. There are a number of papers published that look at this stereotyping and explore when they develop and why. For example a study of occupational therapists (OTs) and nurses in Australia showed that both groups held the other profession in high esteem. However, the OTs were thought to be more interested in intellectual problems and were described as innovative, snobbish, better looking and more likely to have wealthier families while being less well organised, kind and nurturing. Nurses were perceived to be less resistant to change and to gossip more. Both groups rated their own profession as being more interested in people than the other (Westbrook, 2010).

We tend to stereotype professionals' values and approach to patient care as well. An interesting exercise in a mixed group of professionals is to see if you can work out who does what based on their dress, conversation and perceived values. Or to observe different professionals interact with patients and each other and see if there is an obvious professional culture apparent (this task is often foiled by uniforms though).

Jane Day of the School of Interprofessional Health Studies in Ipswich (UK) provides a table of 'values, philosophies and theoretical differences of members of an interprofessional team' (Day, 2006, page 133). While there are certainly some characteristics linked to each profession, I would be cautious of being so certain about these without admitting that there is a certain amount of stereotyping involved. Giving an overarching value to doctors (advocate saving life), nurses (advocate humanism) and social workers (advocate quality of life) is very reductionist and does not take into account the wide variation within the professions. As with patients, we must not assume but explore.

Professional and interprofessional identity

Interesting questions in relation to professional development are how a health professional develops his or her professional identity and how this identification affects his or her working with other professionals. I am also curious as to whether it is possible to identify oneself as having an interprofessional identity. Hammick et al. (2009) titled their book 'Being interprofessional' and suggest that to achieve this health professionals need to have the requisite skills and conduct themselves in the right way with appropriate attitudes, as well as suitable values. However it is unlikely that a person asked 'what do you do' will answer 'I am an interprofessional' rather than 'I am a nurse, doctor, physiotherapist' etc.

Identity has been described as how one defines oneself to oneself and to others (Lasky, 2005). Obviously this definition changes over time and context. So a practice nurse may have referred to herself in the past as a student nurse, then an adult nurse, followed by practice nurse but also on other occasions as a mother; I variously introduce myself as a GP, a health professional educator, a researcher or a medical doctor. The choice is predicated on who asks me and where. Many people involved in health care delivery and education have several job titles, overlapping roles and membership of more than one team – so perhaps we can truly say we are interprofessional or at least interdisciplinary. Thus identity is a continuous process of formation and transformation with individuals continuously constructing and reconstructing their identity because of shifting experiences within their daily lives (Giddens, 1991). This multi-faceted nature of identity means that individuals have to manage competing demands and motivations, which can lead to discomfort, stress, emotional exhaustion and dissatisfaction (Kumar, 2012). One identity framework suggests there are four views of 'what it means to be recognised as a certain kind of person' (Gee, 2001, page 100): the dimensions of nature, institution, discourse and affinity, that are said to be interrelated 'in complex and important ways' (page 101). Gee (2001) contends that these perspectives of identity can be accepted, contested, or rejected in terms of which one dominates in a particular context.

Earlier in this chapter we considered the functionality of teams and the possibility that team members' values may not always be compatible – that there may be clashes of values and furthermore competing values within an individual affected by working with others. In the literature relating to identity this process is called identity dissonance, a term which describes how holding inconsistent or conflicting cognitions (values, attitudes, beliefs) would engender feelings of unease (ie dissonance) that were unpleasant and required resolution (Festinger, 1962). Cognitive dissonance is postulated to be a fundamentally motivational state in that people seek to resolve feelings of dissonance by attempting to reduce the relative importance of the conflicting belief, acquiring new beliefs that lower the dissonance, or entirely remove the conflicting belief. We can substitute value for belief in the previous sentence. In practical terms this means that health professionals working together may be able to adapt their values to resonate with each other's and enable optimal collaboration. However if values and beliefs continue to conflict, one or more of the team may find it difficult to continue to work together.

Costello (2005) has carried out further work on cognitive dissonance in the area of professional identity. Extrapolating from her work regarding law and social work students we can theorise that health professionals' success or failure in their professions is explained by the degree of alignment between their embodied or unconscious self-identity and the views, values, attitudes and behaviours espoused by their chosen profession role. And further that when working interprofessionally alignment between self-identity, professional identity and interprofessional identity is fundamental to collaborative practice.

> **Reflection point**
> How do you identify yourself? Do you relate more to other members of your profession than your team members? Are you interprofessional?

The patient at the centre of the team

I mentioned above the notion that patient-centred care may be thought of as the patient at the centre of the team. For example: 'A care team puts the patient at the centre of the practice with a systematic workflow that is designed from the patient's perspective' (MGMA, 2011). Does this mean the patient is then a member of the team, and what implications does this have for team function? As professionals we would then be in as many teams as we have patients – which does not make sense. The patient at the centre of practice is a more practical way of considering this. We must not let words and definitions get in the way of service. A concept of interest here is 'co-production', which 'refers to the contribution of service users to the provision of services' (Realpe & Wallace, 2010; p8). Co-production challenges the traditional relationship between patients/service users and health service workers, by acknowledging that patients are experts in their own health and circumstances. While the term is often used to refer to co-production of health, it may also be applied to secondary prevention in chronic illness. Particularly for patients with long term conditions, team-based care needs to recognise the patient's expertise and values, and they should where possible be given an equal voice with other team members. In later chapters I return to this idea when discussing shared decision-making and patient choices.

Conclusion

Modern health care is developed and delivered via teamwork and collaborative practice. Team members from different professions will have varying personal and professional values that need to be recognised and discussed for optimal patient/client care. We can learn about how we may work better together from the organisational and sociological literature.

References

Canadian Interprofessional Health Collaborative. (2010). Available at: http://www.cihc.ca/files/CIHC_IPCompetencies_Feb1210r.pdf (Accessed December 2011).

Costello C. (2005). *Professional identity crisis: race, class, gender, and success at professional schools.* Nashville, TN: Vanderbilt University Press.

Dawson JF, Yan X and West MA. (2007). *Positive and negative effects of team working in healthcare: Real and pseudo-teams and their impact on safety.* Birmingham: Aston University.

Day J. (2006). *Interprofessional working.* Cheltenham: Nelson Thornes.

Department for Education and Skills – DfES. (2004). *Every child matters: next steps.* London: DfES.

Department of Health. (2007). *Creating an interprofessional workforce: An education and training framework for health and social care.* London: HMSO.

Festinger L. (1962). *A theory of cognitive dissonance*. London: Tavistock.

Field A. (2009). Diagnosing and fixing dysfunctional teams. Harvard Business Update. Available at: http://www. stoneandcompany.com/uploads/Dignosing%20&%20Fixing%20Dysfunctional%20Teams.pdf) (Accessed October 2011).

Gee J. (2001). Identity as an analytic lens for research in education. *Review of Research in Education*, 25;99–125.

Giddens A. (1991). *Modernity and self-identity*. Cambridge: Polity.

Gittell JH. (2009). *High performance healthcare*. New York: McGraw Hill.

Hammick M, Freeth D, Copperman J and Goodsman D (2009). *Being interprofessional*. Cambridge: Polity.

Institute of Medicine. (2001). *Crossing the quality chasm: A new health system for the 21st century*. Washington, DC: National Academy Press.

Johnson DW and Johnson FP. (2006). Group dynamics. In: *Joining together: group theory and group skills (9th edition)*. Upper Saddle River, NJ: Pearson International.

Katzenbach JR and Smith DK. (1993). *The wisdom of teams: creating the high-performance organization* Boston: Harvard Business School Press.

Kumar K. (2012). Interdisciplinarity in health research: a phenomenological analysis of the lived experience. Unpublished Doctor of Philosophy thesis, The University of Sydney.

Kunzmann C. (2006). *Ontology-based competence management for healthcare training planning: a case study. In: Proceeding of the I-KNOW*. Austria.

Lasky S. (2005). A sociocultural approach to understanding teacher identity, agency and professional vulnerability in a context of secondary school reform. *Teaching and Teacher Education*, 21;899–916.

Lencioni P. (2002). *The five dysfunctions of a team. Lafayette*: The Table Group.

Manion J, Lorimer W and Leander WJ. (1996). *Team-based health care organisations: blueprint for success*. Gaithersburg, MD: Aspen Publishers.

MGMA (2011). Medical Group Management Association. Available at: http://blog.mgma.com/blog/bid/64706/4-steps-to-creating-a-patient-care-team (Accessed January 2012).

Mickan S. (2005). Evaluating the effectiveness of health care teams. *Australian Health Review*, 29;211–217.

Realpe A and Wallace LM. (2010). *What is co-production?* London: The Health Foundation.

Reeves S, Lewin S, Espin S and Zwarenstein M. (2010). *Interprofessional teamwork for health and social care*. London: Blackwells.

Smith S, Nicol KM, Devereux J and Cornbleet MA. (1999). Encounters with doctors: quantity and quality. *Palliative Medicine*, 13;217–223.

Thomson AM, Perry JL and Miller TK. (2009). Conceptualising and measuring collaboration. *Journal of Public Administration Research*, 19;23–56.

Tuckman BW and Jensen MAC. (1977). Stages of small group development revisited. *Group and Organisations Studies*, 2;419–427.

West M and Slater J. (1996). *Teamworking in primary health care: a review of its effectiveness*. London: Health Education Authority.

Westbrook MT. (2010). Professional stereotypes: How occupational therapists and nurses perceive and each other. *Australian Occupational Therapy Journal*, 25;12–17.

World Health Organization. (2010). *Framework for action on interprofessional education and collaborative practice*. Geneva: WHO.

Chapter 3

Communication within teams and between professionals

This chapter explores the nature and importance of communication between health professionals, both those within teams and those working in wider collaborations. We consider how complex communication may be when patient and client care is shared between many professionals. Trust, feedback and the skill to delegate appropriately are essential to optimise communication and collaboration and enhance patient safety. Team meetings and good record keeping are other elements of communication to consider.

The importance of communication between all professionals working with the same patients was highlighted by the now well-known circumstances that occurred in Bristol in the UK, and this case is often referred to as a turning point in patient care. The inquiry into the performance of paediatric heart surgeons in Bristol found that poor communication between different professionals was a factor in the adverse clinical outcomes for the babies involved (Bristol Royal Infirmary Inquiry, 2001). In this hospital setting the professionals may well have identified that they were working in a team, but other recent high profile cases, such as that of Baby P (again in the UK), also show a lack of coordinated care across organisations and failure to discuss concerns by the disparate groups of health and social care professionals and agencies involved.

> **Reflection point**
> What training, if any, have you and/or your team received in communication skills? Consider if such training has been successful and how. What further training do you feel you need?

Health professional students now receive intensive training in communication, primarily to address communication with patients/clients. While teamwork does feature in many health professional curricula, there is less time devoted to the issues of communication between different professionals – from the same and from other professions. Yet 'communication phenomena are surface manifestations of complex configurations of deeply felt beliefs, values and attitudes' (Brown & Starkey, 1994, page 808). Often we offend or misunderstand more from what we do not say as that which we verbalise during interactions. This is not simply about body language but about acknowledgement of diversity and being in tune with our colleagues. As individuals we recognise that we are complicated people, and yet we often presume that we can read and understand our fellow professionals, who are nevertheless as complicated as we are.

The wrong injection

Dr Lynne Marshall is having a bad day. She is running about 30 minutes late with her appointments. Tori Macdonald arrives 20 minutes late for her appointment. Lynne was hoping she would be a DNA (did not attend) but now here she is with her three small children under 5. Tori is 20 and Lynne, while despairing of her patient's life choices, has a soft spot for her and thinks that Tori copes remarkably well with her kids, her errant boyfriend and her lack of money. The children are always clean and fairly polite. Lynne considers telling Tori she cannot see her now because she is so late, but this goes against her professional values. Moreover Tori would need to be seen at some point and might have to be fitted in with one of the other doctors who do not know her so well. Lynne knows that one thing Tori needs is her 3-monthly contraceptive injection (Depo-provera) but also a check on some other problems. To save time Lynne asks Vicky the receptionist if Judith, the practice nurse, could give the 'depo' and that she will see Tori after the next two patients who are waiting.

Twenty minutes later Lynne calls in Tori. Tori has not had her injection. Exasperated Lynne goes into the treatment room. Judith is on her own checking the dressings cupboard, not too busy then Lynne thinks which annoys her even further. Lynne goes to the drug cupboard and finds the 'depo'. Judith asks if she needs the ampoule to be checked. Lynne fires back no and leaves. It is only at the end of the consultation that she realises she has injected Tori with Depo-medrone (a steroid used to treat inflammation) rather than the contraceptive injection she required. 'It's all Judith's fault' she thinks.

In what way is the above scenario about values as well as communication? Let's consider the actors and their possible values:

Tori, is a young mother, and to all extents and purposes a single mum – her children have different fathers. Any judgmental older adults in the waiting room may consider her a waste of space, feckless, getting pregnant because she couldn't be bothered to use contraception or wanted to get a council house, on benefits, and with her children doomed to the same cycle of little education and lack of ambition. In fact Tori, as Lynne knows, is a caring and devoted mother whose children are well cared for by a supportive extended family. OK, Tori may have made some poor life choices (who defines poor?) but she intends to do the best for her kids and her commitment to a long acting contraceptive is a sign that she does not want to get pregnant again anytime soon. She values honesty and would expect Lynne to admit to giving the wrong injection straight away, and would be fine with that, as long as she received the right one today. An unwanted pregnancy on top of everything else would be just too much.

Lynne is a dedicated and empathic doctor with very high standards of care. She is highly involved with her patients and always goes out of her way to provide what she thinks is the best consultation. She values her professionalism and skills and expects the other members of the health centre team to work just as hard and just as carefully as she does. She hates to keep patients waiting, but knows that 10 minute appointments will always lead to her over running, so she is constantly feeling fraught and not at her best. While she values the nurses and works well with them, she does feel that they are in the practice to some extent to take pressure off the doctors, and therefore she expects them to fit in around her own work. They have longer appointment slots (usually 20 minutes) and therefore should be able to see extra patients as necessary. She is stunned by the mistake she has made and thinks it wouldn't have happened if the nurse had been willing to help out: what's the point of the team if she is left to do everything. Injections are more a nurse's work than a doctor's anyway. She is going to be perfectly honest with Tori, of course, but intends to have a few words with Judith when there is time.

Judith is also highly dedicated and proud of her skills. She no longer sees nurses as at the beck and call of doctors (doctors' hand maidens) and enjoys the ability to practise autonomously to some extent. However, she is also keen to help and values the team experience and chance to work with and learn from other professionals. She will always fit in extra patients but only when she has seen her own. She does get miffed if she feels she is being taken advantage of by someone who, realistically, is higher up in the hierarchy. In fact Vicky had forgotten to mention that Tori was waiting to be seen by Judith. Lynne hadn't used the computer messaging service to alert Judith to her request but rather had relied on Vicky who was also flat out on reception. Judith is a stickler for checking drugs; in hospital she has been used to two people checking ampoules and has always felt a bit nervous checking and giving injections by herself. She thinks that Lynne could easily have had her look at the ampoule, especially as the doctors are not as familiar with how the drug cupboard has been recently organised.

There are a number of communication failures present here. The receptionist had not passed onto Judith that a patient was waiting; Lynne had not used the normal method of communicating these referrals between professionals; some of the doctors had not been informed about the rationalisation of the drug cupboard; Lynne had not responded to Judith's offer and Judith has been annoyed by her manner; Lynne and Judith had never discussed how they would like to work together – the manner had just evolved and usually worked quite well until another systems problem intervened. Nurses are trained to check drugs carefully whereas doctors are assumed to check and, because of their greater knowledge of drugs, thought to be less likely to make a mistake (certainly by their own profession).

Unbeknown to either Lynne or Judith, there was also a lack of communication on the part of the receptionist, who had not indicated to Judith that Lynne was waiting, nor to Lynne that Judith also had a full clinic. Vicky, the receptionist, assumed that the two health professionals were using the computer messaging system as outlined to her in her orientation a few months ago. Therefore, in her opinion, there was no need to inform either of them about Tori. In fact Vicky, in a similar situation the previous week, had told Dr Mike Grainger that Judith would like him to check a patient of hers. Mike had said he had already received this message and would act on it when he was free. Vicky had felt he was annoyed at her. Vicky now realises that Lynne's partially disguised anger and Judith's black mood have arisen in part because of her lack of action. She thinks it best though not to say anything.

It is easy to see from all this interplay how a small number of failures add up to a bigger communication issue and ultimately a clinical error. While Tori has been harmed to some extent, the major fallout from this scenario is likely to be strained relationships between these three working women. Such strain may then lead to further problems in the future. I can certainly remember errors I have made when emotionally charged. Hopefully, one or more of them will have a personal value of not leaving work with unaddressed team issues.

Reflection point

How might each individual approach a resolution of this episode? How would you define this teamwork in action? Often we don't discuss our values and ways of working until there is a problem and then, as Tori discovered, it is too late. Though luckily the wrong injection is unlikely to cause her any major harm.

Multiple interactions

In any one day as a busy health professional we will interact with many different people: patients, team members, other staff, our families and friends (Box 3.1). With each person and in each context we adapt the type and style of communication we use, from formal to informal, from professional to lay from complex to simple. The potential for miscommunication is high and yet most of the time we do understand each other. But the evidence is very clear that lapses of patient safety and litigation against health professionals are mainly due to failures of communication. Why do these happen and what part do values have to play in good communication?

Interprofessional communication and communication within teams

Communicating with others is a fundamental human skill, and yet we can get it so wrong so often. Miscommunication, no communication and even too much communication (when confidentiality is an issue) are all everyday problems. One of the underlying factors is lack of time: we are constantly rushing about and while we may try to give patients time, we frequently hurry our interactions with team members and other colleagues. We leave messages rather than pass on information face to face; sometimes these messages are backed up with written notes either in the patient record (likely to be computerised and therefore legible), a message book or on bits of paper (often illegible). I, and I am sure this is not unusual, have not spoken to another GP during a whole morning of consultations; my interactions with the nurses may be to request clinical input or answer a query.

Reflection point

Team building and communication is often facilitated by time to sit and talk together as colleagues about things other than work. How often is there a tea break in your working days now? Or do you ever have lunch together, other than during a work-related meeting?

Communication within our wider circle of collaborators is likely to be via a referral or discharge letter, a phone call or an email. Each method requires particular skills and safeguards. Patients are often reminded of appointments now by text message; text messaging professionals means yet another communication input to check during the day.

A study into communication between health professionals in a UK hospital setting found several examples of inefficiencies with team communication. For instance a senior doctor attempted to transfer a patient between teams by delegating the request through two intermediaries. By the time the receiving specialist was given the message, its meaning had been substantially altered with the potential to affect the patient's safety (Coiera & Toombs, 1998). The authors concluded that individual health professionals must carefully consider the effects

Box 3.1: Some examples of professional communication (adapted from Thistlethwaite and Spencer, 2009)

HP (health professional)–patient communication
- Consultation: face-to-face in a wide variety of contexts.
- Consultation/advice by telephone.
- Written.
- Electronic.
- Use of interpreter.

HP–patient's family/carers
- Face to face (including 'third party' where patient is not present).
- Telephone.
- Written.
- Electronic.

HP–HP (same profession), e.g. doctor-doctor
- Professional, e.g. referral.
- Case discussion.
- Handover.
- Seeking or giving advice.
- Interactions with junior or senior colleagues.
- Appraisal and mentoring.
- Teaching (students and others).
- Treating a doctor as a patient.
- Oral.
- Telephone.
- Written.

HP–HP (different profession), e.g. doctor–nurse
- Referral.
- Seeking or giving advice.
- Consultation in partnership.
- Handover.
- Case discussion.

In teams: conflict resolution and negotiation skills
Running/chairing meetings
- Facilitating a small group educational meeting.
- Practice and interprofessional meetings (multi-disciplinary team meetings).
- Committees.
- Video or tele-conferencing.

Presentations to a large group of professionals
- Lectures
- Case presentations

of their communication behaviour, particularly 'interruptive behaviours', on their own efficiency and effectiveness as well as on that of others.

Interruptions occur all the time in clinical work. They are distracting and can cause a lack of focus and mistakes. Perhaps you have a practice policy about phone calls during consultations, about who can interrupt whom within the team and for what purpose. One professional's value may be that the patient being seen is the sole focus of attention and therefore the professional will not allow phone calls or distractions when a patient is in the consulting room. Others may feel that it is fine to answer the phone if it is a colleague or someone needs urgent advice.

High expectations

I mentioned earlier that Lynne has very high expectations of herself and of others. Maybe we could call her a perfectionist. If team members fall below her high standards, she is apt to get frustrated and even angry. She is aware of this – she often gets annoyed on the phone when dealing with organisations, which have failed to give her 'adequate' service. She feels that if she worked in this way, she would soon receive a complaint. When affronted, she tends to talk too much and complain about what has been done, rather than accept the problem and look at ways to rectify it. Her communication skills with patients are exemplary, but with others not always so. She is always mortified when she has lost her temper (though she never swears) and is actively trying to be calmer in these situations. How does she communicate this value to members of the team?

If she says 'I always expect the best from my colleagues', they might say they do always do their best. The problem isn't the willingness, but the definition of best. Expecting perfection as the only meaning of best is likely to cause disappointment and bad feeling. Moreover, if Lynne doesn't feel she will get the best, she is liable to take the job on herself and perhaps not do it so well or she may become burnt out through an excessive workload.

A key skill for professionals is the ability to delegate. Delegation of a task to another means that we have to trust the person to do the job properly, at the right time and for the right person. Learning to delegate can be difficult if you are a perfectionist and cannot trust anyone to do a job as well as you would. If you have the value that task delegation is in fact an abdication of responsibility, then you are going to have problems. Moreover, teamwork is about dividing tasks and ensuring that the most appropriate person has the most appropriate tasks to perform. A perfectionist is going to find it difficult working within a team. She will constantly be checking on the jobs and may frequently state 'I should have done that myself, it would have saved time'.

Task delegation requires good communication in terms of what must be done and when, how much leeway there is and what the expected outcomes are. Handover is a form of delegation, though it is rarely called handover in community settings. One team member may be finishing a shift, going on leave or taking on new roles. It is important to hand over patient care and tasks with the right amount of information: too much and it will be difficult to assimilate; too little and errors are likely.

Poorly performed handover may put patient safety at risk and can lead to poor continuity of care, adverse events and even litigation (Wong et al., 2008). Examples of information that may need to be transferred and acted upon when someone is away are: results of investigations, home visit follow-up of sick patients; telephone check following a new prescription etc. Face-to-face handover is obviously safer but needs to be backed up with written records. Verbal handover only, compared to verbal handover with some written notes, relies heavily on memory and is therefore a high risk strategy (Bhabra et al., 2007). If carried out face-to-face or via telephone, written notes should be made about what has been said, what instructions given and agreed goals. Having a practice agreed strategy with perhaps a handover template and computer reminders, with spaces for appropriate information, ensures that the correct information is given and retained.

> **Reflection point**
> What system does your team or workplace have for handing over information? Is it reliable? How might you improve the process?

Feedback

In the scenario Lynne and Judith are left with negative feelings about their colleague. Rather than take these to a practice meeting to discuss with the whole team, they could agree to give each other feedback on what could have been done differently to avoid a similar situation in future. Once they have sorted out their grievances, they can present the issue of the wrong injection to the whole team as a significant event analysis (see Chapter 4), so all can learn without apportioning blame.

In addition to the features of high performing teams already discussed in Chapter 2, we can add the ability for team members to give and receive feedback, because they feel safe and trust one another, and the team has the value of facilitating open communication. Many educators will have experience of learning to give feedback to students particularly feedback in relation to patient interactions. A framework commonly used in medical training for role play, work with simulated patients and work-based consultations is what is now referred to as the Pendleton guidelines (Box 3.2). These are rather formal and time consuming for the needs of Lynne and Judith, but giving positive feedback in conjunction with discussing what could be done differently in future is a good method for being fair.

> **Box 3.2: Guidelines for feedback – adapted from Pendleton et al. (1984)**
> - Clarify any points of information/fact.
> - Consider what you and your colleague did well – ensure that you identify the strengths of the communication and do not stray into weaknesses.
> - Discuss what went well and how to build on this.
> - Consider what went less well and what you would/could do differently next time.

Thus Judith could say to Lynne: 'We obviously had a problem earlier. I could see you were having a difficult session and I was pleased you thought I could help. Normally I would have been able to manage Tori but you had forgotten to send me a message about her waiting. Usually the messaging system works well and that really is the best way to let me know if you need me. I am glad that the mix-up with the injection wasn't serious. It is so rare for you to make a mistake. I am happy to check injections anytime and I will speak to the other nurses about improving the storage of the injections so that similar ones are not kept side by side'. And Lynne could say to Judith: 'I am sorry I was annoyed earlier. I realise that I should have sent you a message about Tori. You are always so helpful when I'm under pressure. I will remember to use the computer to send you the message next time. Perhaps you could also see if there is a patient waiting outside the treatment room for you if you are free. It can sometimes be difficult to send messages when I'm busy and maybe we need to review this system at a meeting. I will also talk to Vicky about passing on patient requests'.

Team meetings for business

In chapter 2 we saw that regular team meetings are vital for team functioning. Members need to be committed to meeting (rather than thinking, oh no not another meeting!) and therefore meetings should be productive, well led and keep to time.

A regular meeting slot at similar time intervals is essential for core meetings: once a week, once a fortnight or whatever is appropriate. For extended team meetings, such as professional development sessions, the day of the week might be rotated to allow people to attend more often. But for core business, a set day, time and place are more helpful so that diary reminders can be set up annually. Meetings should start and finish on time. There is an art to deciding how much business to include in a meeting so it does not over run. Getting to know team members and being able to handle both the verbose and quiet participants are key skills for those acting as chairpersons. Meetings should not last more than 2 hours and their location should be such that everyone can be comfortably seated with a clear view of all present. The chair of the meeting may always be the same person, depending on the circumstances, and is often the practice manager in a health centre. However the chair could be rotated to ensure that all professions have a chance to take on this role.

A staff member should be designated as the meeting secretary, to help compile the agenda and send it out in good time. People need to know what will be discussed, as well as the standing items, so they can be prepared with any necessary material. While core meetings may be a place for discussion, it is imperative that they produce decisions and outcomes and that people feel they have a say in these outcomes. Agenda items need to be labeled as for: exploration, information, decision, and/or action. Those items that result in action need to be logged with the team member responsible for that action and the date by which there will be an outcome.

Reaching a decision may be easy or may be quite difficult depending on how well the possible courses of action resonate with or against team and individual values. When there are several options the team needs to consider the advantages and disadvantages of each. This is a similar process to a shared decision making approach with a patient, but the team as a whole and as members need to be considered. The team may have agreed a way to reach consensus: this may involve a vote, a final decision by the leader after hearing all the discussion, or no option being chosen unless there is agreement by everyone (consensus).

Of interest here is the relative power of the various health professionals involved and the type of environment in which they are working. In a general practice partnership in which everyone apart from the doctor partners are employees, the power obviously lies with the doctors, but that power may not be exercised except in certain circumstances, perhaps affecting the financial stability of profits of the 'business'. In a primary care organisation or other health centre, where everyone is a salaried employee, doctors may still have the power because of their status, but may not in fact have the final say in what happens, particularly if money is involved.

Meetings to discuss patient/client cases

These are a specific type of meeting to discuss patient management (patient complaints and errors will be dealt with in Chapter 4). Depending on the professionals involved in the patient's care, there might need to be an agreement about what the patient is called: client, service user or perhaps just by name. An interesting discussion is, if the team has declared a value which defines the patient as at the centre of the team, whether the patient and/or carer should be present at these meetings.

Meetings to discuss individual patients are necessary when there is a complex problem and an extended team, but probably are not so vital if team members can discuss patients while they are being treated. These meetings are often referred to as multidisciplinary team (MDT) meetings, and one aim is to help programme a patient's journey through the health care system, ensuring that all the appropriate professionals play an active role in management (Day, 2006). As discussed earlier when thinking of the difference between 'inter' and 'multi', it is important that the professionals work together and communicate, rather than working side by side without agreement. MDTs are commonly formed in cancer care, palliative end of life care and child protection. Team members need to be committed to meeting during their busy schedules and may have to travel if not co-located.

In the past I found as a busy GP that child protection meetings were often held at short notice and in a morning when I was booked into a surgery, which was invariably full. So doctors were often the professionals missing from the discussion and our knowledge of the family and children was often relayed by a letter or phone call: not ideal. The result of the meeting was then communicated by another letter or phone call. MDT meetings are time consuming but as well as helping coordinate care, provide an opportunity to meet other professionals face to face and to learn about roles and responsibilities.

Clinical notes

How many sets of notes does a patient like Tori have? She has her general practice records (computerised), her hospital notes from her deliveries (likely to be paper), perhaps others at the local child health clinic and yet a fourth set with social services. There will be duplication of some letters across these various records, but each volume contains different information, in different words and with different emphases. There should be processes in common though (Box 3.3).

Box 3.3: The clinical record

- Clear and succinct notes.
- No abbreviations unless agreed and with similar meanings across professions.
- No jargon.
- No insulting language.
- Legible writing if hand written.
- Dated and signed unless computerised.
- Contemporaneous as much as possible.
- Changes initialled and dated.
- Write what you would be happy for others, including the patient, to read.
- Record what information you have given the patient.
- Would the next person reading the notes understand what has happened and what is going to happen.

There needs to be a clear practice policy on who can read what in a patient's notes – and this policy needs to be communicated to patients. Patients often think that all health professionals are connected electronically and that their histories and drug records are available almost instantly. This misconception sometime means that they do not want certain information recording as it might be read by people other than the person in whom they are confiding.

Assertive behaviour within teams

Most of us will be aware of the distinction between the desirability of being assertive and the impropriety of being aggressive. Assertion is the right to express one's own ideas and values while at the same time respecting those of the other person. The psychological literature defines assertion as a skill that can be learnt. It is an expressive skill, involving verbal and non-verbal communication, and it entails risk: risk that the recipient may react negatively in the interaction (Rakos, 1997).

Examples of assertive behaviour in a team context is a team member declining a request to do a task that she feels unable to do or has not time to do. A less assertive person might agree to do the task because she does not want to admit a lack of skill or because she does not like to let people down. The outcome might be that the task is performed poorly or not at all, causing more problems in the long run. But some professionals are unable to say 'no', and certainly not to someone they perceive as superior. When thinking of a response to such a request, there are four elements to consider (Box 3.4).

> **Box 3.4:** Assertion response elements (from Rakos, 1997)
> - Content: What the person says or replies.
> - Paralinguistic elements: How the person says it (tone of voice, loudness etc).
> - Non-verbal cues: Body movements, stance, facial expression, gestures, touch.
> - Social interaction skills: Timing, persistence (e.g. if a request is repeated).

Of interest here, in view of Lynne's demands for perfectionism both in herself and her colleagues, is that research has shown that irrational ideas like this (or in this case her values) are more likely in non-assertive people. Rakos (1997) gives an example of a typical thought process [and meaning] to illustrate this:

'I must assert myself without any mistakes or the assertion will fail [self-perfection], the other person will think I'm a jerk or will be hurt or angry [universal approval], and that would be absolutely terrible [catastrophising]. It would be my fault [self-blame] and confirm that I am no good [self-denigration]. It will be work out better if I let it pass and see what happens [inaction]' (page 307).

Rakos (1997) suggests other thought processes or rational alternatives, which may be learnt. These include acceptance of imperfection, acceptance of disapproval (you cannot satisfy everyone all the time), non-catastrophising (things rarely turn out as badly as you think – for example taking a day off work for sickness is unlikely to cause your whole practice to run to a halt), taking appropriate action and enhancing self-worth.

Conflict: negotiation and resolution

The positives and negatives of conflict within teams were touched on in Chapter 2. Conflict may lead to innovation once resolved but also continuing animosity between members if allowed to fester (Jehn, 1995). There has been a lot of research into team conflict particularly as reported in the organisational and business literature. One systematic review suggested that overall conflict has a damaging impact on team outcomes (De Dreu & Weingart, 2003), which intuitively seems likely if we consider our own experience. Unfortunately even within health care teams there is bullying and discrimination. In health care team terms this impact is probably going to have an effect on patient care, and possibly professional job satisfaction and retention.

> **Reflection point**
>
> How would you give feedback to a team member or colleague following an episode of poor communication? How would you deal with the issue if you had been at fault?

A few thoughts about patient safety

Good communication is essential for patient safety; poor or miscommunication often results in adverse events. One definition of patient safety is the reduction of risk of unnecessary harm associated with health care to an acceptable minimum (Runciman et al., 2009). The WHO has stated that patient safety is a fundamental principle of health care, and thus a core value, and that at every point in the process of care-giving there is a certain degree of inherent unsafety (WHO, 2011). For patients with complex needs who interact with a high number of health professionals, there are patient safety issues relating to communication (Schoen et al., 2009). The percentage of adverse events due to communication is difficult to quantify, as communication is often an additional factor in such problems as passing on investigation results and medication errors. The National Patient Safety Agency in the UK (NPSA) has published 'Seven steps to patient safety' which are summarised in Box 3.5. In terms of reporting, learning and sharing, one suggested method is the SEA (significant event analysis), which is discussed in Chapter 4.

> **Box 3.5:** Seven steps to patient safety (NPSA, 2009)
>
> 1. Build a safety culture.
> 2. Lead and support your practice team.
> 3. Integrate your risk management strategy.
> 4. Promote reporting.
> 5. Involve and communicate with patients and the public.
> 6. Learn and share safety lessons.
> 7. Implement solutions to prevent harm.

> **Reflection point**
>
> What do you understand by patient safety? Is patient safety as a concept discussed within your team? What resources do you know of that you could use to enhance team function in this area?

Conclusion

There is no doubt that communication is one of the major factors to ensure optimal team functioning and collaborative practice. Communications skills may be learnt and it is vital that health professionals uphold the value of personal interaction and respect to enhance patient safety.

References

Bhabra G, Mackeith SPM and Pothier DD. (2007). An experimental comparison of handover methods. *Annals of The Royal College of Surgeons of England*, **89**;298–300.

Bristol Royal Infirmary Inquiry. (2001). *Learning from Bristol: the report of the public inquiry into children's heart surgery at the Bristol Royal Infirmary 1984–1995.* London: Stationery Office. Available at: www.bristol-inquiry.org.uk/ (Accessed September 2011).

Brown A and Starkey K. (1994). The effect of organisational culture on communication and information. *Journal of Management Studies*, **31**;807–828.

Coiera E and Tombs V. (1998). Communication behaviours in a hospital setting: an observational study. *BMJ*, **316**;673–676.

Day J. (2006). *Interprofessional working.* Cheltenham: Nelson Thornes.

De Dreu CKW and Weingart LR. (2003). Tack versus relationship conflict, team performance and team member satisfaction: a meta-analysis. *Journal of Applied Psychology*, **8**;858–866.

Jehn KA. (1995). A multimethod examination of the benefits and detriments of intragroup conflict. *Administrative Science Quarterly*, **40**;256–284.

National Patient Safety Agency. (2009). Available at: www.nrls.npsa.nhs.uk/resources/collections/seven-steps-to-patient-safety/ (Accessed December 2011).

Pendleton D, Schofield T, Tate P and Havelock P. (1984). *The consultation: an approach to learning and teaching.* Oxford: Oxford University Press.

Rakos F. (1997). Asserting and confronting. In: Hargie GDW (Ed). *The handbook of communication skills. (2nd edition).* London: Routledge. p289–319.

Runciman W, Hibbert P, Thomson R, Van Der Schaaf T, Sherman H and Lewalle P. (2009). Towards an international classification for patient safety: key concepts and terms. *International Journal for Quality in Health Care*, **21**;18–26.

Schoen C, Osborn R, How SKH, Doty MM and Peugh J. (2009). In chronic condition: experiences of patients with complex health care needs, in eight countries, 2008. *Health Affairs (Millwood)*, **28**;w1–16.

Thistlethwaite JE and Spencer JA. (2009). *Professionalism in medicine.* Abingdon: Radcliffe Medical Press.

Wong MC, Yee KC and Turner P. (2008). *Clinical handover literature review, eHealth Services Research Group, University of Tasmania Australia.* Available from: http://www.safetyandquality.gov.au/internet/safety/publishing.nsf/Content/PriorityProgram-05 (Accessed September 2011).

World Health Organization. Available at: www.who.int/topics/patient_safety/en/ (Accessed December 2011).

4

A patient complaint: team meetings, policy and practice values – raising awareness in the team

This chapter explores the issues surrounding a patient's complaint about his treatment at a general practice (family medicine) surgery/clinic. We consider the importance of good medical record keeping, team meetings, establishing practice values and the role of significant event analysis (SEA) in patient care.

It is Tuesday evening and the City Health Centre in the north of England is busy as usual. There are two GPs (one male and one female) and two nurses (one female practice nurse and one female advanced nurse practitioner) seeing patients through a mix of booked appointments (for registered patients) and as walk-in patients (who wait in a 'queue' to be seen). This health centre is both a traditional general practice surgery with registered patients and a walk-in centre for people requiring acute but not emergency health care. Walk-in patients do not need to be registered at this practice; they attend the centre because they are unable to wait for a consultation at their own registered practice.

David Turner is a 49 year old registered patient who rarely attends the surgery. Tonight he arrives without an appointment at 6pm and asks to see a doctor, preferably male. The receptionist informs him that the only available slot is with the nurse practitioner, who will be able to see him in about 20–30 minutes. David reluctantly agrees to this and takes a seat. From his position he has a clear view of the reception area and over the next half an hour sees practice staff coming and going, including a man he concludes is one of the GPs. This person is chatting to the receptionist for at least 10 minutes; it is difficult to hear what is being said; however, there is quite a lot of laughter. A young woman with a baby comes in and asks to see a GP, and the presumed male doctor agrees to see her there and then. Eventually, after 40 minutes, David is called through to see Susan Wright, the experienced nurse practitioner. David informs her he has had bleeding from his back passage for the last week on and off, and presumes he has a recurrence of the piles that troubled him about 2 years ago. Susan asks him some questions and then suggests she examines him. David is not keen on this, and says he would prefer a male practitioner. Susan therefore suggests that yes, it is possible he has piles, that she can prescribe some cream but that it is important he sees a doctor if the problem persists. David again asks if he could see the male doctor on duty, the one who was in reception earlier. Susan says this is not possible as the doctor is busy and the surgery will be closing shortly. David takes the prescription and leaves. Two months later he makes an appointment to see a different male GP, who questions and examines him. Dr Barrett says that David requires further tests to exclude more serious problems than piles.

David is eventually diagnosed with bowel cancer, which is treated at the local hospital. He writes a letter of complaint to the practice manager about his care: his inability to see a GP when required, his management by Susan, the behaviour of the receptionist and the subsequent delay in his diagnosis. The letter is discussed at the next practice meeting to decide on a reply.

> **Reflection point**
>
> What are your immediate reactions to this story? Consider your own viewpoint based on the bare details given above: how might this be affected by your profession, your own experience of attending a surgery as a patient and your experience of complaints (one against you or perhaps dealing with one against a colleague, or your workplace in general). How is your viewpoint coloured by your values? Is there anyone for whom you particularly feel sympathy or empathy? Or anger? What other emotions do you have and why?
>
> Now think about the team in this narrative. How would you describe the functioning of the team? What evidence is there of teamwork?

Initial thoughts on this scenario

There are a number of people involved in this story, all of who would narrate the events in different ways, depending on their role within them, their values, expectations and emotions. Their stories would also probably differ if they were asked to recount them on that first evening or after the complaint was received. Health professionals and patients reading the story will also have different ideas on what was happening and what might be done better, depending on their backgrounds and values.

I am sure you would want more information about the evening. The story as written is mainly from David's perspective, as is the letter of complaint. What might he and the other actors in this drama be thinking?

The patient's perspective

[Note: I am writing this from my position as a health professional, therefore can I ever really espouse a patient's perspective? As health professionals we may try to put ourselves in the shoes of the patient, perhaps bringing to this attempt our own experiences of seeking health care. But there is always a large gap between what we know and how we are treated by our colleagues, and what lay people (for want of a better word) know and how they are treated. Having said that we can attempt to surmise David's thoughts and values and, as the narrator here, I have the power to decide what these might be.]

I rarely attend the surgery because I feel healthy most of the time, I find the opening times inconvenient because I work long hours and also I prefer not to be poked and prodded. However I do know that the bleeding I have been having could be a sign of something sinister at my age (I have read stuff about screening for bowel cancer and how common the condition is). I still really think it is piles as I have had these before (or at least that was what I was told by a GP a few years ago – he examined me but didn't do any tests). I really want to see a male GP and it seems to me that women are allowed to choose to see women doctors (my wife always insists on this), so there should be a male doctor for me. I would just feel more comfortable. I think male doctors are more matter of fact and I don't want to discuss anything other than my symptoms. I expect, like last time, I will need an examination, that's ok if there is no fuss.

I did feel lucky to get an appointment. I hear a lot about the difficulty of getting in to see a doctor. My wife was also concerned and she said that our surgery now has a walk-in centre. I am not entirely sure what this is but it suggests that you should be able to see someone if you walk into the surgery. I know that this bleeding is not an emergency (so I wouldn't go to casualty/emergency department) but I don't want it to go on unchecked without seeking advice. I did feel disgruntled that I could only get an appointment with a female and a nurse at that. I am not confident that a nurse will be able to sort out my problem (nurses do injections and dressings) and I presume I will need a further consultation with a doctor, wasting more time. The receptionist was quite offhand. She said the nurse is a nurse practitioner, but I don't know how that is different, and when I asked what that meant, she said the nurse was more experienced (more experienced than what?). I was surprised the nurse offered to examine me, but did not want this because she was female and because I expected a doctor would have to repeat the examination later, and who wants a finger stuck up there more than once? I felt fobbed off by the whole experience – as if a cream will sort things out. I didn't return straight away as the experience was unpleasant – there was a doctor available in my opinion, who would have been better seeing patients rather than laughing with receptionists. And how come that other woman walked in and was seen straight away? I also couldn't get into the surgery for a while because of work commitments. Being told I had bowel cancer made me even more angry, and I want some explanation about why I was left to see a nurse. And brooding over this even more, I wonder if the bowel cancer was present at my original consultation 2 years ago – never piles at all.

The patient's ideas, concerns, expectations and values

If we now adopt a patient-centred perspective on the story, again bearing in mind that we are not patients in the same way, we could make a list of David's ideas, concerns, expectations and values. In terms of the ideas, concerns and expectations (ICE), these may and often do change depending on the circumstances. His values, however, will be more static, and they will influence ICE. David has the idea that he has piles, but he is concerned it may be more serious (cancer) and he expects to see a doctor, be examined and managed appropriately. Now think of his possible values and compare to the following list.

Values

- I should have the choice of gender of my health care professional.
- If I think my problem is urgent, I should be able to be seen the same day.
- I do not think that people should say a problem is urgent just to be seen straight away if it is trivial.
- By urgent I do not mean life threatening but bleeding at my age is urgent.
- I should not have to go into great detail about my problem in order for a receptionist to take me seriously.
- Doctors should put their patients first.
- Only doctors (not nurses) can deal with certain problems such as those that need a diagnosis.
- I shouldn't have to repeat my story to more than one person at the practice.
- I shouldn't have to be examined by more than one person at the practice.

- The doctor should be able to make a diagnosis and refer me quickly for further treatment if I have certain symptoms.
- If I complain, I should be taken seriously.

David's complaint, like most complaints, is precipitated by a failure of the system (in this case the general practice clinic and its staff) to engage with his concerns, to meet his expectations and/or to gel with his values. If we consider the practice staff now we can see how their values may conflict with his. Each member of staff is likely to have personal, professional and possibly practice values.

Practice values and the mission statement

Speaking of 'the practice' we need to consider what we actually mean. The practice is made up of the staff working within it but also the patients and community it serves. Does your practice have 'values'? Maybe you have a practice mission statement or a statement of goals and objectives. Mission statements were all the vogue a decade or so ago but the term is not used so much now. A business world definition and explanation is given in Box 4.1. Here the emphasis is on purpose, products and services. The word 'ideals' is used rather than values.

Box 4.1: One perspective of the purpose and development of a mission statement

'A mission statement is a statement that defines the essence or purpose of a company – what it stands for i.e. what broad products or services it intends to offer customers. The mission statement also gives readers a window on the **raison d'être** of the company and was initially designed as a means by which potential shareholders and investors could understand the purpose of the company that they were considering investing in. You should also think of a mission statement as a cross between a slogan and a mini *executive summary*.

Just as slogans and executive summaries can be used in many ways, so too can a mission statement. An effective mission statement should be concise enough for you to *describe your company*'s purpose and ideals in less than 30 seconds.'

An effective mission statement is best developed with input by all the members of an organisation.

The best mission statements tend to be three to four sentences long.

Avoid saying how great you are, what great quality and what great service you provide.

Examine other company's mission statements, but make certain your statement is you and not some other company. That is why you should not copy a mission statement.

Make sure you actually believe in your mission statement. If you don't, it's a lie, and your customers will soon realise it.

From: http://articles.bplans.co.uk/writing-a-business-plan/mission-statement/367 by Alan Gleeson (Accessed December 2011).

A general practice may have an agreed policy rather than a mission statement. Consider the questions in Box 4.2. How many of these are you able to answer? (Note I use mission statement, policy and vision as similar terms – you may call this concept something else.)

Perhaps in David's practice there is a policy that patients will be seen on the same day if they have an 'urgent' problem, but that this is unlikely to be with the doctor or nurse of their choice. If there is no doctor available, they will be offered a consultation with a nurse practitioner or practice nurse, depending on the problem. This means that the patient has to give the receptionist some idea of symptoms so she can make a judgement. Should this

---

Box 4.2: The practice mission statement

- Who was/is responsible for formulating the practice vision/mission statement?
- How does the mission statement feed into or reflect practice policy?
- How involved was the community (for example the patient participation group) in setting the vision? How often is this and/or policy reviewed?
- Does everyone agree with the mission statement?
- How is it communicated to new staff and to new patients?
- What values are enshrined in this policy?
- Are there any conflicts with personal or professional, team or patient values?
- How would you know?

---

be the role of a receptionist? In some practices, this triage will in fact be carried out by a nurse. The practice may also prioritise in terms of age: for example children under 10 always seen the same day without exception, patients over 70 given priority.

Practice staff may have agreed this policy but might not have considered it could conflict with patient expectations. Moreover patients are not always aware of the roles and responsibilities of the members of the health care team and may not value an appointment with a nurse as highly as one with a doctor. On the other hand, some people prefer to see a nurse for certain conditions – nurse appointments are often longer; some patients may not be as in awe of nurses as much as doctors; nurses may be viewed as more caring.

Reflection point

Patients and professionals will have different opinions as to what is 'urgent'. What would you classify as urgent from a **medical** perspective? From a **nursing** perspective? Does one's profession make a difference to the definition? It is almost certainly different from the lay perspective. In your experience what do patients mean by 'urgent', 'acute' and 'emergency'?

Urgent suggests that this is a problem that cannot wait until tomorrow, that the patient's condition is such that he or she will deteriorate overnight unless treatment is given. Urgent for a patient might be more related to an anxiety about causation, or a change in symptoms, or something that is uncomfortable but not life threatening. Patients may have had symptoms for a few weeks but something happens that makes them want help now. The patients' concerns define urgency; their values dictate what should be available to resolve the problem. There has been a great deal written about people's inappropriate use of emergency departments for non-urgent problems in many countries around the world (see for example Hoot & Aronsky, 2008). The causes are multiple and complex. The establishment of walk-in centres in the UK was partly in response to this problem, but reports from 2004 and 2007 failed to show any improvement (Cooke et al., 2004; Salisbury et al., 2007).

In terms of gender, we have accepted for some time that women patients should have the choice to have a female doctor. This is much more likely these days as the gender balance at medical school is more equal. In fact there is more of a risk of there being a lack of male GPs in the future. It is rare for practices to be single gender and indeed women may choose to register only at practices where a female is available. Nurses are still predominantly female within community settings, and patients may expect a female rather than a male nurse. Similarly there are still very few male midwives yet very many more male obstetricians. We have to accept that some men are more comfortable seeing a male doctor, and when arranging appointments, the gender of the doctor (or other health professional) should be stated for both male and female patients. However, we might think it unreasonable for a same day appointment to be offered with the preferred gender of professional.

So it is acceptable to want a choice of professional by gender. However it is not acceptable to want a choice by race. A practice is unlikely to acquiesce to a request by a patient to see the 'white doctor'. Is it acceptable to request an appointment with a professional who is a native English or a native Punjabi speaker? Perhaps we are prepared to work within the parameters of some values but not others.

Making a complaint

All general practices in the UK should have a complaints procedure according to the NHS website for patients: *NHS Choices. Your health, your choices* (Box 4.3).

Box 4.3: GP complaints

'All GP surgeries should have a written complaints procedure, and you will find this at reception or on the practice website.

- As a first step, speak to the practice manager. You can also complain to the practice in writing, or by email.
- If this doesn't resolve the problem, or you'd rather not raise the issue directly with the practice, you can complain to the local primary care trust (PCT).
- The NHS Constitution explains your rights when it comes to making a complaint.

You have the right to:

- Have your complaint dealt with efficiently, and properly investigated.
- Know the outcome of any investigation into your complaint.
- Take your complaint to the independent Parliamentary and Health Service Ombudsman if you're not satisfied with the way the NHS has dealt with your complaint.
- Make a claim for judicial review if you think you've been directly affected by an unlawful act or decision of an NHS body.
- Receive compensation if you've been harmed.'

From: http://www.nhs.uk/choiceintheNHS/Yourchoices/GPchoice/Pages/GPcomplaints. aspx (Accessed December 2011).

Reflection point

Have you ever had a complaint against you or your practice or workplace? How did you feel? Several different combinations of emotions may arise: anxiety, anger, doubt, guilt, why me? Even relief if the complaint is about one of your colleagues and not yourself. When you know more about the circumstances, even though your notes and reflection lead you to conclude that you have no cause to feel alarmed, you will still feel anxious.

In this scenario David is complaining about a number of factors and several people. The letter has been addressed to the practice manager (Emma Caldwell) who will instigate a review. First, however, she will acknowledge receipt of David's letter and give him some idea of the complaints process: how she will investigate and how long before he hears anything further.

She might also ask for clarification at this point if there are missing data such as the date of the incident.

The doctors' perspective

'If Mr Turner was so concerned about his bleeding he wouldn't have left it so long to return for another appointment.'

This statement by one of the GPs is a defensive remark – he is trying to deflect possible blame from himself or the practice by putting the onus on the patient to seek appropriate care, and thus is indirectly blaming the patient for the outcome. He is also attributing to David his, the GP's, own value of the necessity, indeed the imperative, to seek help in a timely manner and that this is the patient's responsibility. Other examples of such remarks could be:

'I advised the patient to come back for the results in a week, but he didn't return until his symptoms got worse, 3 months later.'

'I told the patient to stop taking the pills if they made him more dizzy, but he kept on taking them and that caused him to fall off the ladder.'

'He'd had the symptoms for 3 months and then insisted on an urgent appointment.'

Of course people do have responsibilities for their actions but health professionals need to be aware that people as patients are often vulnerable, anxious and confused, their health literacy (Box 4.4) may be low and they may not hear or understand the professionals' advice or management plan.

Box 4.4: Definition of health literacy

Health literacy is the degree to which individuals have the capacity to obtain, process and understand basic health information and services needed to make appropriate health decisions (US Department of Health and Human Services, 2000).

The nurse practitioner's perspective

Susan Wright is identified in the practice leaflet as a nurse practitioner though the preferred term in the UK is advanced nurse practitioner. There is certainly confusion about the role and responsibilities of these health professionals, as evidenced by David's uncertainty. The Royal College of Nursing (RCN) in the UK defines an advanced nurse practitioner as a registered nurse with a university honours degree and who 'makes professionally autonomous decisions for which he or she is accountable' (RCN, 2010, page 3). Thus Susan can consult with patients with undifferentiated and undiagnosed problems, may undertake a physical examination, order investigations and prescribe medication. Susan is covered with indemnity insurance by the RCN.

Reflection point

How does your practice or how should a practice describe to patients what the roles and responsibilities are of the health professionals who work there? If you are not a nurse practitioner yourself, are you fully cognisant of this role?

This is the first complaint that Sarah has been involved with. While she is able to practise autonomously she works within the team environment and is able to ask for advice if unsure of what to do. She feels aggrieved that David did not respect her professionalism and competence, but she is used to being considered at the same level of expertise as a practice nurse. She considers that she advised David to be followed up and she did consider the possibility of other causes of his rectal bleeding, but felt he needed to be examined before deciding on referral or otherwise. As she knows that many doctors are not happy that nurse practitioners are undertaking some of the doctor's traditional tasks, she feels vulnerable to criticism and wants to stand up for her profession.

The effects of the complaint

At the time of receiving a complaint it is best not to try to attribute blame to anyone but to investigate the circumstances including what has happened, the personalities involved and the emotions raised. In larger organisations, such as hospitals, different professional groups may blame each other rather than taking a systems approach to seeking causation:

'If the doctors would only listen more to patients.'

'Since nurses began getting university degrees, they spend less time with patients and neglect their basic nursing needs.'

And in clinics where other practitioners are involved: 'The physiotherapist should have read the notes and seen that the patient couldn't do that exercise.'

Alternatively to becoming defensive, the professional may be overcome with guilt, justified or not, simply because of receiving a complaint. If a professional has a low self-esteem, or on-going personal or professional difficulties, they may react badly to a complaint and find it difficult to continue working. They may wish to apologise to the complainant just to make the complaint go away. While we no longer think that professionals should not apologise under any circumstances, as this was thought to be an admission of guilt, at this stage in the story the apology is best delivered in terms of the whole practice while not apportioning blame until the circumstances are investigated.

How might Emma respond to the letter in the first instance?

A good start is:

Dear Mr Turner

I would like to acknowledge your letter of the 6th June. I am very sorry that you feel that you have received unsatisfactory treatment at the practice. I will be looking into the issues you raised …

Interprofessional aspects: evolving roles and responsibilities

Dr Bridgman is the most senior of the partners and is due to retire in the next year. He was never keen on employing a nurse practitioner (NP), though he was very happy with the work of the practice nurses. In his mind only doctors are trained to diagnose and then prescribe. NPs were fine for following protocols in such areas as contraception and asthma, but new symptoms like rectal bleeding should always be dealt with by a doctor. He was therefore not surprised that Mr Turner had complained and, whatever the outcome, would like this incident to stimulate a practice discussion about the role of the nurses in the health centre. Dr Bridgman also feels that general practice is becoming more consumer driven. He did accept the need for a walk-in centre but does not like the way that patients, in his words, abuse the system and now feel they can access medical care at any time and for any reason.

Importance of contemporaneous notes

Health professionals have some advantage in providing evidence of what has happened in terms of the patient record: IF they have recorded the relevant facts. However the record is never a complete transcript of what happened but is an interpretation of events. While there may be common elements relating to symptoms, examination results and management plan, the details of the conversation and what has been understood by the patient is missing; after all the notes are made by the professional not the patient. Moreover, what happens outside the consulting room is not recorded (unless on CCTV which is not common), so often deciding on what happened comes down to what people remember, who is thought to be more likely to be correct and what is written in the notes.

Do the notes of different professionals differ? Even with a template to fill in, we decide on what is important. There is inter and intra-professional diversity in note keeping. Often there are even separate sets of records that each profession keeps – though usually within general practice there is one computerised record. However community nurses have separate documents.

> **Reflection point**
>
> Has your practice discussed what should be in records? Do you audit their quality – and indeed have you defined what is meant by quality? Do you ever give feedback to a colleague because a patient's notes were excellent or poor?

The practice meeting

Practices usually hold regular meetings to discuss complaints and this may be through a significant event analysis (SEA) process (also known as significant event audit). A significant event is any event thought by anyone in the team to be significant in the care of patients or the conduct of the practice (Pringle et al., 1995). A patient complaint is obviously significant and this one seems to involve a possible missed diagnosis of cancer, a lack of patient choice and inappropriate management. A number of members of the practice team are also implicated.

According to the UK National Patient Safety Agency (NPSA): 'Improving the quality and safety of patient care is a key clinical governance priority in primary health care and SEA has an important role in contributing to this aim' (NPSA, 2008 online). A SEA should involve all members of the practice team, learning from each other and contributing to the discussion.

A SEA has seven stages (adapted from the NPSA website), which relate to the values-based concepts of mutual respect for differences of values and balanced decision making within a framework of shared values.

Stage 1 – A staff member becomes aware of a significant event and makes it a priority for a practice meeting and discussion. In this case the practice manager receives the complaint and tables it for the next meeting. Her staff are familiar with this type of audit and by having a set routine for management of events, they should feel more comfortable about discussing the problems, without a blame culture being adopted.

Stage 2 – Before, if possible, and also during the meeting, information needs to be collected and collated from all personnel involved. David's computer records need to be scrutinised, including his previous consultation for 'piles' and his medical history. Are the records sufficient to give a good idea of what happened during the consultations? Obviously there will be no written records of this request to see a male health professional or what went on in the waiting room.

Stage 3 – The facilitated team-based meeting is the important step in allowing discussion, and in this stage any difference in personal and professional values may become apparent. There needs to be a decision about who will facilitate the meeting – not a person who is directly involved in the complaint. The practice will already have set ground rules for this type of meeting, but the facilitator needs to remind the team of these. Discussion should be open, honest and non-threatening. However everyone needs to be aware that emotions may be difficult and that the aim of the meeting is not to apportion blame but to explore what has happened and to learn from this, in order to prevent an occurrence in the future. Of interest is that the patient is not present at these discussions, nor might there be any patient perspective other than the complaint letter.

Stage 4 – To analyse the significant event the team needs to be able to ascertain: what happened on the day that David attended the health centre; why circumstances unfolded as they did; what should be learnt from the events and what, if anything, needs to be changed. SEA may be explored in this way without an actual complaint but because a member of staff has identified a problem. In David's case the results of the meeting also need to be reported to him. This might be best done face-to-face with the practice manager and/or one of the more senior clinical members.

Stage 5 – The agreed action should be implemented by staff designated to co-ordinate and monitor change. The NPSA suggests that one way of testing how well the process has been carried out is for the team to ask: 'What is the chance of this event happening again?'

Stage 6 – The meeting needs to be written up. A person, other than the facilitator, should be taking minutes and these should include a record of any action points and who is responsible for these. The minutes should be circulated to all staff in confidence.

Stage 7 – Report, share and review – the practice should formally report (either to the National Reporting and Learning Service, or via the primary care trust/ health care organisation) those events where patient safety has, or could have been, compromised.

Potential outcomes of the meeting

The meeting identifies a number of areas that need to be discussed and action taken. These include providing further information to patients about on-the-day appointments and what they are for, the scope of practice of each of the different health professionals and how this information is shared with all the staff and the patients.

The team also talks about follow-up consultations for potentially sinister symptoms. There is a well organised system for reviewing test results and ensuring that patients who do not return for results within a limited time frame are contacted. But patients with symptoms are usually advised to return if they do not clear up within a certain time. The onus is on the patient to contact the surgery. The team agrees that in this case David should have been made an appointment to see one of the male doctors within the week for further assessment and examination. All agree it is better to be pro-active than risk missing a diagnosis. How far the patient should be chased if they do not come back is debated for quite a while. The consensus view is then that patients do have autonomy and should take responsibility if they are given and understand all the facts and uncertainties about their underlying conditions.

Within the hierarchy of professional roles all agreed that ultimately, while uncertainty remains about a diagnosis, and if there are risk factors for potentially serious conditions, a doctor should see the patient, but that this should not undermine the role of the advanced nurse practitioner in diagnosis and treatment of more minor problems.

Emma and the last doctor to see David arrange to meet him to discuss the issues. He is happy that his complaint was taken seriously and that changes have been made to practice protocols. He decides not to take the matter any further and continues to attend the practice.

Lay commentary

Reading this chapter as a lay person, my sympathy is with the patient, David Turner. Mine was a fairly emotional response, perhaps fuelled by the general air of 'mystique' which patients often feel about their GP's practice, despite information being more readily available via the Internet than ever before.

David's own values, and his embarrassment, precluded him from being examined on that Tuesday evening visit, and, in my opinion, a more sensitive receptionist should have made the male doctor aware of the situation, then a completely different scenario may have ensued. Similarly, the nurse practitioner was not made aware of David's reticence to see a female health professional on this occasion, but could still have spoken to the male doctor when an examination was refused.

Many patients feel that their practice surgery is shrouded in mystery, and have no notion of the roles of the surgery staff, with the exception of the GPs, who are qualified to deal with their health problems. David has no understanding of what difference there is between a practice nurse and a nurse practitioner, and, like him, I have no notion of how far a receptionist's responsibility extends and how much authority they should be given to enquire into the nature of a patient's complaint, or indeed, what they are instructed to do when they have ascertained that information. Are they given instructions or guidelines for such an occasion, or are they purely using their own values to arrive at a decision?

David started this scenario 'on the back foot' as soon as the receptionist asked him what was wrong with him. This is an all too familiar story, when receptionists are perceived as gatekeepers employed to 'weed out' malingerers. There appears to be a distinct lack of team work at this practice, it is difficult to understand why the receptionist, the nurse practitioner and the male doctor could not briefly communicate with each other while the patient was still in situ.

The analysis of the scenario is very thorough, however I would add these points:

- In addition to the practice mission statement, an explanation of the role, expertise and authority of every member of staff would save anxiety for many patients, and could be issued to each new patient, and made available for existing patients, although it would not necessarily change David's preference to see a male doctor.
- Many companies display a 'who's who' board in their reception, showing photographs and job titles of their staff – this may be a helpful addition in a surgery reception/waiting area.
- When a patient complains to/about a practice, are they informed of the SEA procedure? Or do they simply receive a letter from the practice manager saying 'we'll look into it'?

- As a patient, I would welcome the opportunity to actually voice my opinion, perhaps in a one to one meeting with the practice manager before the SEA process, which seems to preclude my involvement.

These points do not deal, however, with an 'over-zealous' or 'rude' receptionist. I would suggest that the principles of a practice ensure that reception – the first contact for the patient – is staffed by well-trained individuals and that the principles create a strict set of guidelines by which the reception staff operate. They must also 'buy-in' to the practice mission statement. Looking at my own GP's practice, I am not at all sure that the receptionists are trained in anything other than the computer system.

We all form our opinions and derive our values from the information provided to us. David's information is incomplete, and a potential situation of this nature might be averted with more clarity and transparency from the practice.

> **Reflection point**
>
> What are your reactions to the lay commentary? Do you feel you need to change anything about your practice after reading this chapter?

Conclusion

We have explored a number of themes arising from this scenario some of which related more obviously to values-based practice than others. There is an underlying theme of communication here as well, verbal and written, that needs to be considered. Every practice will received complaints; how these are dealt with reflect the values of the team.

References

Cooke M, Fisher JD, Dale J, McLeod E, Walley P and Wilson S. (2004). *Reducing attendances and waits in emergency departments. A systematic review of present innovations. Report to the National Co-ordinating Centre for NHS Service Delivery and Organisation.* Available at: www.sdo.nihr.ac.uk/files/project/SDO_ES_08-1204-029_V01.pdf (Accessed December 2011).

Hoot NR and Aronsky D. (2008). Systematic review odf emergency department crowding. *Annals of Emergency Medicine*, **52**; 126–136.

NPSA. (2008). Available at: www.nrls.npsa.nhs.uk/resources/?entryid45=61500 (Accessed December 2011).

Pringle M, Bradley CP, Carmichael CM, Wallis H and Moore A. (1995). *Significant event auditing. A study of the feasibility and potential of case-based auditing in primary medical care.* Occasional Paper No. 70. Royal College of General Practitioners. London: RCGP.

RCN. (2010). Advanced nurse practitioners – an RCN guide to the advanced nurse practitioner role, competences and programme accreditation. London: RCN. Available at: www.rcn.org.uk/__data/assets/pdf_file/0003/146478/003207.pdf (Accessed December 2011).

Salisbury C, Hollinghurst S, Montgomery A, Cooke M, Munro J, Sharp D and Chalder M. (2007). The impact of co-located NHS walk-in centres on emergency departments. *Emergency Medicine Journal*, **24**, 265–269.

US Department of Health and Human Services. (2000). *Healthy people 2010.* Washington, DC: US Government Printing Office.

Chapter

5

A well person health check, health promotion and disease prevention: different lifestyles, different values

This chapter considers the meaning and nature of health and what it means to be healthy, the utility and value of check-ups for health and well being, including screening tests. We work through different scenarios relating to check-ups in primary care.

Tuesday afternoon and it is the monthly clinical practice meeting, which is attended by all the clinical staff (GPs, nurses, the pharmacist and the counsellor), plus the practice manager, Megan Daly. At the Station Road practice there are a number of special clinics for patients with specific health needs and problems: diabetes, asthma, cardiovascular risk, family planning, travel clinic. The nurses also check the health of the over 75 year age group.

Dr Steven Reynolds has asked the practice team to discuss well person checks and what these should involve based on evidence. He says he was asked by a 35 year old man for a check-up in a 10 minute appointment. When he asked the patient if he had any particular concerns about his health, the man replied that no he just wanted a 'going over' to make sure he had no hidden illnesses, 'you know, like those private health checks they advertise in magazines, an MOT'. Dr Reynolds admits to feeling irritated by this request. MOT after all stands for Ministry of Transport and refers to a roadworthy assessment of a vehicle, not a human being. Private health checks are an expensive waste of time in his opinion. Moreover he points out that the cardiovascular risk assessment is offered to the over 45s in the practice and carried out by the practice nurses. What does everyone think about other check-ups? Ann Lorimer, the most senior practice nurse, says that all patients should be able to have a health check if they request one: what should be done in this would depend on their age and family history. Women were used to coming in for smears, from their twenties, and would be asked about smoking and other lifestyle choices, so why not offer something for the men to encourage them to attend for advice about healthy living.

> **Reflection point**
>
> At this point consider the possible values of Dr Reynolds, Ann Lorimer and the patient that impact on this scenario. What do you feel about check-ups and why? Do you offer them to patients? What are their values?

Thinking about check-ups – the practice discussion

Dr Reynolds first asks – what do we as health professionals mean by check-ups? Are they the same as a well person health check, a new patient consultation or what we used to call well woman checks? How do check-ups fit in with screening or risk assessments? The difference might be related to whether a person is asymptomatic or has certain symptoms requiring diagnostic tests. Dr Reynolds suggests that they think about the requests they have for check-ups and consider whether they fit the criteria for screening in the World Health Organization's list of requirements for screening (Box 5.1). Screening is for very specific conditions such as sexually transmitted infection particularly chlamydia; in contrast risk assessment uses a combination of factors, such as lifestyle, family history and physical examination, together with risk tables to give a percentage risk of developing a condition, most commonly cardiovascular disease.

Box 5.1: Criteria for screening tests (Wilson & Jungner, 1968)

Screening: aims to detect a disease in an individual without signs or symptoms.

- The condition should be an important health problem.
- There should be a treatment for the condition.
- Facilities for diagnosis and treatment should be available.
- There should be a latent stage of the disease.
- There should be a test or examination for the condition.
- The test should be acceptable to the population.
- The natural history of the disease should be adequately understood.
- There should be an agreed policy on whom to treat.
- The total cost of finding a case should be economically balanced in relation to medical expenditure as a whole.
- Case-finding should be a continuous process, not just a 'once and for all' project.
- The test should be sensitive (few false negative).
- The test should be specific (few false positives).

The Station Road GPs rarely get involved in screening or risk assessment these days. Cervical smears and blood pressure checks are usually carried out by the nurses unless, for example, the woman is symptomatic or the patient's blood pressure has been raised on several occasions. The doctors do insurance medicals but tend to find them tedious and of low value, except for the monetary gain. There is a feeling that it is the 'worried well' who ask for check-ups: patients who have read about diseases and are anxious about contracting them or having them. These patients may have symptoms, but not symptoms that add up to give an obvious diagnostic pattern. Dr Reynolds feels that the worried well are over investigated 'just in case'. The inverse care law is still valid (Box 5.2).

Box 5.2: The inverse care law

'The availability of good medical care tends to vary inversely with the need for the population served. This…operates more completely where medical care is most exposed to market forces, and less so where such exposure is reduced' (Hart, 1971).

The inverse care law was defined by Dr Julian Tudor Hart, who worked as a GP in the same Welsh mining village for many years.

Megan Daly suggests that one course of action is to ask the patient why they want a check-up. Ann replies that this question would have to be carefully worded so as not to sound as if the clinician is irritated and as if the request is a waste of time. 'But it is in most cases' says

Steven. There is an obvious difference of opinion between the health professionals of the value of individual patient-professional interactions around prevention through risk assessment and screening. Steven in particular compares individual intervention unfavourably compared to public health measures and media information such as health messages on cigarette packages. Megan intervenes. 'Let's think about why a 35 year old man, let's call him Paul, might ask for a check-up'.

> **Reflection point**
> Why do patients ask for check-ups? Consider any recent requests: did you ask the patient why do you want a check-up now?

Paul might ask because:

- He wants to be pro-active about his health as he gets older.
- He thinks that there are male check-ups similar to that which his girlfriend has – she says she is going for a check-up when she makes an appointment for a smear.
- His friend's firm has paid for senior staff to have private medicals.
- He is going to join a gym and he has been told he should consult a doctor first.
- He has a specific worry due to family history, friend's illness or something he saw in the media.
- He has a specific symptom but doesn't want to mention it to start with.

Now let's think why some of us don't see the value in this for Paul:

- We are assuming he has no symptoms.
- We are biased against the worried well.
- The inverse care law preys on our minds.
- We know the evidence for certain types of screening.
- We know that mass screening of low risk people for certain conditions is not cost effective.
- We know that examining asymptomatic patients is unlikely to reveal anything serious.
- But also that it sometimes can.
- An unforeseen physical sign in an asymptomatic patient may require investigation and management that is ultimately more harmful than the condition diagnosed.
- We know that many physical signs don't correlate with serious pathology.
- We believe that there can never be a totally 'normal' check-up.
- Most risk tables do not include the under 40 age group.
- Telling a patient you have found nothing wrong may prevent them returning with new onset symptoms.
- Telling a patient you have found nothing wrong, does not mean there is nothing wrong with them.
- Telling a patient you have found nothing wrong, may not prevent their continuing to worry.
- If you find nothing wrong but use the consultation for lifestyle advice such as anti-smoking and safe limits for alcohol, patients may not feel as motivated to change 'as there is nothing wrong'.

Perhaps we can compare a 'check-up' with a cardiovascular risk assessment:

- The risk assessment is based on evidence from numerous studies.
- It is fairly quick and simple to do (though Ann points out this depends on what is found and any counselling that is required, and many patients do not fully understand what risks as percentages mean).
- Most of the assessment relates to social history/lifestyle and family history.
- There is evidence that changing behaviour actually reduces risk, e.g. stopping smoking, losing weight.

There is now an interesting discussion about how evidence changes. For example, in August–September 2011 there were conflicting opinions in the British Medical Journal as to the role of salt in hypertension (Graudal & Jürgens, 2011; Cappuccio et al., 2011). These messages, often distorted, get into the media: 'It is no wonder that patients get confused – the advice is always changing' says Ann in frustration. As part of risk assessment and secondary prevention the nurses routinely advise against adding extra salt to the diet.

There are other check-ups we need to consider that have as part of their rationale screening for potential problems: antenatal and post-natal, well baby, child development, sexual health (STIs), the over 75s and skin checks (these more common in Australia for example). That is before we step deeper into controversy with more specific tests such as prostate specific antigen (PSA) and mammograms in younger women.

There is also a dark side to the culture of check-ups. Professionals may be paid for doing these and then we need to ask if the financial gain changes the value of a check-up in their eyes. Do they still think they are a waste of time or do they really believe they have the potential to improve people's health and morbidity and reduce mortality? Do our values change in line with secondary gain, or only our behaviour? And we can excuse our behaviour by saying it is what the patient wanted anyway and the patient was prepared to pay.

So, in summary, what we are saying is:

Professionals need to explore with patients the reason for asking for a check-up:

- What do patients think a check-up entails – what is being checked?
- What do they want to find out?
- And why?
- What will they do with the information?
- Are they prepared to change behaviour if necessary?

Other questions

If we do check-ups, we need to decide how often, what age groups, when to start and, possibly, when to stop. A useful resource for helping to answer some of these questions is the Red Book published by the Royal Australian College of General Practitioners – latest 7th edition published in 2009, but likely to be updated in 2012 (RACGP, 2009). There are some differences with UK policy (again raising questions of the use of evidence, for example age to start screening for cervical cancer and frequency – in the UK start at age 25 then every 3 years; in Australia start as age 20 and then every 2 years) but the data are all captured in one place.

Health, wellness and being normal

The more we think about the nature of a check-up, the more complex may become the reflections on language. If we consider that a check-up is to check on the state of someone's health, do we then conclude that it gives us an answer as to whether someone is healthy or not? Which then begs the question as to what is meant by health and healthy. If we are healthy, are we well? One of our values may be to make every effort to keep healthy. Other people may have the value to get as much enjoyment out of life as possible, including indulging in risky behaviour such as illicit drug use, extreme sports and unprotected sexual intercourse.

> **Reflection point**
>
> How do you measure health? Would you say you were healthy? There are differences in what is thought of as risky behaviour. Does your team agree on what is risk and how to counsel patients about this?

A quick exercise would be to ask the staff of Station Road Surgery how they would define health and healthy. Is there likely to be much difference between the health professions, and then between the professions and the 'lay' staff? We might then ask a patient…

The WHO constitution (1948) defines health as: 'A state of complete physical, social and mental well-being, and not merely the absence of disease or infirmity'. Today we could also add spiritual well-being. Using this definition we might be hard pressed to think of anyone who is in a state of health. If we further consider health as an abstract state, then being healthy is a very subjective opinion. It would be hard to devise a series of assessments that could measure physical, social and mental well-being objectively – that all people being assessed would agree with. Deciding oneself, or someone else, is healthy is very much a value judgment. We can use the types of measures available to health and social care practitioners such as vital statistics (weight, body mass index, blood pressure), mental health surveys and standard of living indices, but these may fail to give an holistic picture of someone's state of being. As health professionals we should have a great interest in what constitutes health and our role in not only promoting health but also ensuring that our communities have the potential to achieve health in terms of those other factors that are important. The Ottawa Charter (1986), which views health as a fundamental human right, emphasises that there are certain prerequisites for health. These include peace, adequate economic resources, food and shelter, and a stable eco-system and sustainable resource use. In terms of values, we would also add freedom from persecution for having diverse value systems and lifestyle choices. Which of these do we, or our patients, have control over? Which do we campaign for in the name of social justice?

So, should our check-ups include an exploration of the social and the spiritual? We probably attend in some measure to physical and mental. The spiritual is more controversial. Recently a GP in England received a warning from the General Medical Council not to give religious advice to his patients (BBC, 2011). The GMC has given guidance to doctors about the discussion of their own and patients' personal beliefs in consultations (Box 5.3). Therefore asking about spiritual beliefs may be open to interpretation.

Illness is usually easier to define than health, though often we consider it in the negative: illness is the absence of health, 'I am **unwell**'; though being unhealthy does not necessarily mean illness. Defining someone as being in the state of 'being ill' can be objective or subjective, whereas saying that someone has a disease or is diseased is an objective process, through

---

Box 5.3: Personal beliefs and medical guidance for doctors (GMC, 2008)

'You should not normally discuss your personal beliefs with patients unless those beliefs are directly relevant to the patient's care. You must not impose your beliefs on patients, or cause distress by the inappropriate or insensitive expression of religious, political or other beliefs or views. Equally, you must not put pressure on patients to discuss or justify their beliefs (or the absence of them).'

---

diagnosis. I may be ill if I have certain physical signs (e.g. raised temperature, rash, enlarged liver etc), but I may also be ill without external or internal signs that can be found by blood tests, radiology etc. Illness may be diagnosed by my history, my symptoms, mine and my doctor's interpretation of my symptoms, and then at some point it becomes a disease. I may say 'but I feel ill' when the doctor says 'I can find nothing wrong with you'. This is then often translated by the patient into 'I can find nothing physically wrong with you'. So then I understand that the illness is in my mind – and may think that the doctor believes I am either mentally unwell or that I am making things up.

When giving the results of a check-up, the professional is advised to say all the tests show normal results, rather than that the patient is healthy: there could be something hidden away that we haven't yet found. Can we truly say this patient is healthy? We might be able to say they are in good health.

Risk taking

Risk is the possibility of suffering harm or loss from an action or behaviour and the chance that a hazard will give rise to harm. We all know of people who are risk takers, who thrive on adrenalin, and those who are risk adverse, preferring to leave nothing to chance. Health professionals need to have skills in discussing risk – not only the risk of an illness, investigation, treatment or non-treatment, but also the risks of certain types of behaviour. How we frame the risk may depend on our own attitudes to risk and our own values relating to particular risks. Discussing risk with patients assumes that they will want to make rational decisions but their health beliefs, values and personal experience may lead them to make choices or carry on with a lifestyle that seems irrational to health professionals (Thornton, 2003). Short term gain from say illicit drug use or binge drinking of alcohol often motivates a person more than the long term health benefits of abstaining from such behaviour (Tversky & Kahnemann, 1981).

Reflection point

What if any risky behaviour do you indulge in? How may this affect your discussions with patients about their risks? Consider the mixed messages that people may receive from the practice team members if they have different values in relation to certain risks.

Check-ups for chronic conditions

The increasing prevalence of chronic diseases and conditions such as diabetes, hypertension, ischaemic heart disease and asthma has prompted many GPs to set up special clinics for monitoring patients with these conditions. Many such initiatives also attract funding, which helps make them attractive over and above the professional value of wanting to help patients stay as healthy as possible considering their condition. Clinics work on the principles of secondary prevention – ensuring that people with health problems do not develop secondary conditions from poor management of their primary disease. Another rationale is that one or more team members can become more specialised in certain areas and that patients with specific conditions can be invited in at the same time for those professionals to use their extra capability. The danger is that patients then become labelled with their disease: the diabetic patient, the asthmatic patient, rather than the patient with diabetes or Miss Smith, who has asthma.

Chronic conditions often benefit from teamwork so that a patient with diabetes attending the practice diabetic clinic may see a doctor, a diabetes nurse, a podiatrist and a nutritionist at the same visit. But does the team work interprofessionally? Do they meet before, during or after the clinic to discuss optimum patient management? And if they do is the patient present?

> **Reflection point**
> Do you run special clinics in your workplace? Consider the professionals involved. Do they work as a team? Is the patient considered to be part of the team? How are patient goals set?

We would define multiprofessional teamwork in the common scenario as the patient interacting with each team member consecutively and being given a list of advice from different perspectives. Such advice may indeed be conflicting. In contrast, if the team is interprofessional, the patient may be seen by two or more professionals at the same time, with the professionals conferring on the best management plan in partnership with the patient. If there is the potential for conflicting advice, there is time and space to discuss, compromise and negotiate consensus. In the best scenario, the professionals also learn from and about each other: about different professional values, evidence and approach.

A patient with diabetes

Connie Ashgrove is a 75 year old woman, who was diagnosed with type 2 diabetes 8 years ago. Her diabetic control is variable and her weight also fluctuates. She had a right total hip replacement for arthritis 3 years ago and has symptoms and signs of arthritis in both knees. She was widowed last year and now lives alone apart from her cat. Both her sons live some distance from her home but one visits her about once a month.

Today she attends the practice diabetic clinic and first sees practice nurse Angela Thomson. Since her last clinic attendance three months ago, Connie's weight has gone up by several kilos (she asks for this to be translated into pounds). Her BMI (body mass index) is 30, her blood pressure is 154/94 and her Hb1Ac (glycosylated haemoglobin) is 8.4% (advised to be lower than 7%). Overall these figures tell the story that her underlying condition and diabetes control are not good. Angela tells Connie that the doctor will probably want to change her medication and that she needs to speak to Sarah, the dietician, who is also in clinic. Connie has heard this all before. She is fully aware that she is overweight. She is regularly advised to do more exercise, but that is difficult given her sore knees and the fact she lives on a hill. She does get out; luckily there is a bus stop nearby while her son also gives her money for taxis for the shopping or she sometimes has it delivered. The dietician has given her a meal plan, but it doesn't include her favourite foods, and she is not that interested in cooking anything fancy. Connie is used to disappointing the health professionals who try to manage her health.

The above scenario is very common. Patients with multiple risk factors, polypharmacy (Connie is on six drugs and likely to get another for her continued hypertension), social issues and biomedical targets for blood sugar, blood pressure, weight etc, take up a lot of the primary care team's time and energy. The nurse and the GP want to see Connie's blood results get better, her weight and blood pressure reduce and, therefore, her life expectancy increase. The dietician and the podiatrist, who will also talk to her today, work within similar parameters, though the podiatrist does ask Connie about her walking and understands that her living environment mitigates against her proposed exercise regimen. These values resonate with those of wanting to help patients' health improve. Yet, perhaps we professionals don't always look at the broader picture of health and quality of life.

If we were to observe the various interactions of the clinic, Connie moving between the four professionals, we notice that they do all give the same message and all have similar goals for Connie. They use different words and have different emphases, but the overall message is diabetic control, weight loss, healthy diet and drug compliance. The last is important, especially to the doctor, the prescriber, as some of the problems could be related to Connie's not always taking her medicine as prescribed. If she does, she needs yet another antihypertensive, if she doesn't she needs the message reinforcing that SHE MUST TAKE HER TABLETS EVERY DAY.

However, today something different is happening in the clinic. There is a final year medical student from the local medical school present and Dr Joy, the GP helping to run the clinic with Angela, asks her to have a chat to Connie about her diabetes and medical care. Jodie is an excellent student and, like many of her generation, has received excellent communication skills training during her programme. Jodie is also a naturally warm person who likes the company of the elderly. She does sometimes find it difficult to 'clerk' patients in the time allowed (which can be anything from 10 to 45 minutes). While Jodie has a good grasp of the aetiology, prognosis and management of diabetes, she is still exploring its manifestations in different patients. She considers the patient before the blood results. After introducing herself (and asking if she may call Connie 'Connie'), she starts with a very open invitation: 'please tell me about yourself Connie and why you are at the clinic today'.

Can Jodie, a fairly healthy, health professional student, of normal weight, who does not have diabetes and is on no prescription medication put herself into the shoes of Connie and really understand what her life is like? Jodie is certain to ask Connie about her ideas about diabetes, her concerns and her expectations of treatment (ICE), following the patient-centred approach she has learnt in her communication skills training. She is unlikely to ask about her values in so many words but asking one or more of the following might lead to a values-based discussion:

- What does living with diabetes mean to you?
- What would you like to change about your health?
- What do you think you could change about your health?
- What do you most enjoy in your daily life?
- What would you find hardest to give up?

Thus ICE becomes ICE-StAR: ideas, concerns, expectations plus exploring the patient's strengths, aspirations and resources.

Let's suppose that Connie is very honest. She may well be to Jodie, this young, enthusiastic and interested young person. This is not to say she lies to the other health professionals, just that she doesn't say what she is really thinking. Connie says that just for once she would like someone to say well done, or be more positive in terms of her achievements. It always seems to be the same message of the need to cut down, need to lose weight, need to exercise more, need to take your medicine properly. Connie really does know all this but it isn't easy. Eating is one of her pleasures in life, but not cooking. What else is there to do for the next 5 years? Connie wants to know why everyone is so obsessed with her blood sugar – after all it is much better than what it was 8 years ago.

As a medical student Jodie has been well primed in terms of evidence-based practice but has also realised in her short medical career so far that evidence is not static and that new evidence is being published regularly. She has also noticed in her time spent with physicians and at diabetic clinics that patients' blood results are often treated rather than the patient (Jodie is a reflective and perceptive student). Her recent reading of the British Medical Journal has changed her mind somewhat about the value of intensive blood sugar control, but she is unsure how this should be applied to Connie's situation. A meta-analysis showed no benefit of intensive treatment to lower blood glucose on all cause mortality and deaths from cardiovascular causes in adults with type 2 diabetes. The authors concluded that therapeutic escalation should be limited and intensive glucose lowering considered with caution (Boussageon et al., 2011). Given that Connie is already on the highest dose of metformin, is taking a sulphonylurea that is likely to be hindering any weight loss, and does not herself want to take any more pills, is trying to reduce her Hb1Ac even further classified as 'intensive lowering'?

Health professional students value becoming members of the team when they are learning in clinical environments. Jodie is able to discuss Connie's ideas and values with the rest of the team in the clinic, who endeavour to take these into consideration when planning further care.

Reflection point

How often do you step outside the parameters of medical care and consider the patient behind the test results? Is there a difference between the professions in terms of considering a patient holistically rather than as their disease? Consider also what health professional students add to your workplace – do they see things in a different light?

Lifestyle choices and values

Jenny Hudson has been a nurse practitioner for 3 years. Her working life has been dominated by impending budget cuts to health services, withdrawal of some services from NHS treatment and a greater scrutiny of her referrals to secondary care to reduce inappropriate out-patient visits. She is a nurse with a high sense of service and wants to do her best for patients, while recognising the constraints and need to ration services (though no-one refers to the changes as rationing).

At a practice meeting she asks the team to consider two of her patients. Max is a 63 year old man with intermittent claudication who has been smoking 15 a day since his teens. He requires vascular surgery in order to save his right leg. Maureen is a 77 year old with complications from her diabetes. She also has poor circulation in both legs and needs referral. She is a non-smoker. Jenny asks hypothetically if only one person could receive treatment, who would it be and why? 'If we are commissioning services and only have a certain amount of money, how do we make these choices?'

Reflection point

What would you say? Who should make these values judgments and how?

But now let's add into the equation: Max is in middle management at the local factory and has no plans to retire as yet. He is of average build and married with two children and four grandchildren. Maureen has been a housewife for most of her life, occasionally working as a dinner lady or shop assistant. Her BMI is 31 and her eyesight is poor. She is widowed and has three children and five grandchildren.

Within health professional circles there is now a certain stigma attached to smoking as a lifestyle choice. While few health professionals now smoke themselves, some do. Are they likely to be more sympathetic to a younger man who smokes than an older woman with other risk factors relating to lifestyle? One set of values: smoking is a legal activity and cigarettes generate revenue through tax. We cannot judge patients on the aetiology of their illnesses otherwise we wouldn't treat sports injuries, obesity, alcohol or even sexually transmitted diseases if people chose not to wear condoms. Where would it end? Moreover we cannot say that smoking is morally or ethically wrong. Another set of values: no one is forced to smoke and most people are fully aware of the risks of smoking. It might be addictive but people need to want to change and many don't. They put pleasure before their health and therefore why should we spend health services money on treating them if they intend to carry on smoking and therefore reduce the benefits of any intervention?

Breast examinations in asymptomatic women

Chiara Vasquez is a 23 year old biology student from the USA who is undertaking a Masters degree. She attends the student medical practice one morning and asks for an appointment with a doctor for a well woman check. The receptionist says that she can see one of the practice nurses for this but Chiara says she wants to see a doctor, preferably a gynaecologist. Eventually she is seen by practice nurse Alison Petrie. Chiara says she is due for her annual Pap (cervical) smear and breast examination. Is the nurse qualified to do these?

Reflection point

What are your feelings here and what might be the potential clash of values? Consider the evidence for this type of screening and think how you may interact with Chiara.

Chiara has been told, like many Americans, that annual examinations are necessary. This has now become her value in terms of seeking good health. She understands that the British system is different in terms of public services and imagines that examinations are performed less often for reasons of costs not health. Alison imagines that examinations in the USA are performed more often for reasons of costs not health – doctors must be making quite a lot of money performing unnecessary intimate examinations. Alison is also a bit aggrieved at having her skills questioned – she carries out the majority of smears for the asymptomatic women, but the practice does not routinely do breast examinations for asymptomatic patients. She wonders if she should advise Chiara about the evidence.

As health professionals we may judge people who do not look after their health, but we also judge those who become 'obsessed' with their health, or in this case potential ill-health. People pick and choose which screening tests and check-ups to have depending on media messages and such like. If, in some jurisdictions, professionals encourage annual physicals, then we cannot blame our clients from continuing to look for a similar level of service in future. Withdrawing an established test is as difficult as introducing a new one.

Clinical breast examination for asymptomatic women has not been shown to reduce mortality from breast cancer, though it may increase morbidity due to unnecessary further investigations including biopsies (Thistlethwaite & Stewart, 2007). The general advice is that women should be breast aware and see their health professional if they notice any changes in their breasts including, of course, lumps. It is very hard however to deny a woman a breast check if they request one. And, of course, occasionally a clinician will find a previously unnoticed lump in a woman's breast, which will affect how they view such requests in future. In a given group practice the doctors and nurses may have different views on the utility of breast examinations, and indeed other tests. Can there be a practice consensus on such matters so that patients do not receive mixed messages?

Conclusion

This chapter has only touched on some of the issues relating to screening, risk and prevention. It is an area with an extensive evidence base but also one that is intertwined with personal and professional values in relation to that evidence and choice. There are no easy answers to many of the questions raised. Reflecting on the issues and discussing them with colleagues, the work team and patients may help resolve dilemmas for individuals. Team-based discussion of evidence usually aims at consensus: 'let's see if we can agree on the evidence'; team-based discussion on values acknowledges diversity: 'let's agree to disagree'.

References

BBC. (2011). Available at: www.bbc.co.uk/news/uk-england-kent-15021419 (Accessed November 2011).

Boussageon R, Bejan-Angoulvant T, Saadatian-Elahi M, et al. (2011). Effect of intensive glucose lowering treatment on all cause mortality, cardiovascular death, and microvascular events in type 2 diabetes: meta-analysis of randomised controlled trials. *BMJ*, **343**;d4169.

Cappuccio FP, Capewell S, Lincold P and McPherson K. (2011). Policy options to reduce population salt intake. *BMJ*, **343**;d4995.

General Medical Council. (2008). *Regulating doctors, ensuring good medical practice.* Available at: www.gmc-uk.org/guidance/ethical guidance/personal beliefs.asp (Accessed November 2011).

Graudal N and Jürgens G. (2011). The sodium phantom. *BMJ*, **343**;d6119.

Hart JT. (1971). The inverse care law. *The Lancet*, **297**;405–412.

Ottawa Charter. (1986). Available at: www.who.int/hpr/NPH/docs/ottawa_charter_hp.pdf (Accessed November 2011).

RACGP. (2009). *The Red Book* (7th edition). Available at: www.racgp.org.au/Content/NavigationMenu/ClinicalResources/RACGPGuidelines/TheRedBook/redbook_7th_edition_May_2009.pdf (Accessed November 2011).

Thistlethwaite JE and Stewart RA. (2007). Clinical breast examination for asymptomatic women: exploring the evidence. *Australian Family Physician*, **36**;145–150.

Thornton H. (2003). Patients' understanding of risk. *BMJ*, **327**;693–694.

Tversky A and Kahnemann D. (1981). The framing of decisions and the psychology of choice. *Science*, **211**;453–458.

Wilson JMG and Jungner G. (1968). Principles and practice of screening for disease. Geneva: WHO. Available at: http://whqlibdoc.who.int/php/WHO_PHP_34.pdf (Accessed November 2011).

World Health Organization. (1948). *World Health Organization Constitution*. Geneva: WHO.

Chapter

6

A patient with medically unexplained symptoms: applying evidence and values for shared decision-making, self-care and co-production of health

This chapter explores the difficulties of diagnosis and management of patients with unexplained symptoms and what has been referred to as psychosomatic illness. The scenario draws attention to the working relationship of a practice nurse and a GP, as well as the value of experience in consultations of this type.

The personal trainer

Andrew Norton is a 29 year old personal trainer (as recorded in his notes). An extremely fit looking young man thinks Dr Paula Chang as Andrew enters the room. Dr Chang is however surprised to see that this is Andrew's sixth consultation in the last few weeks. In his first consultation he complained of strange feelings in his arms, then intermittent headaches, followed by aching hands and feet, and two episodes of chest pain, lasting about 5 minutes. He has seen two of the other GPs in the practice about these symptoms. Both had elicited fairly full histories and carried out focused physical examinations. Andrew had then had some blood tests (all normal). The notes from his last visit state that he was concerned about having a serious physical illness. Dr Smith has written: 'Pattern of symptoms not conclusive. Possibly excessive exercising. Denies steroid use. Medical certificate for one week; advised to rest and then review'. For some reason Andrew has not chosen to see Dr Smith again. Dr Chang wonders if this is because Andrew is not happy with the way he has been dealt with. She wonders if Andrew has now chosen to see the female doctor who has a reputation in the community of being more empathic.

> **Reflection point**
>
> Consider the above scenario – a very typical primary care story. What assumptions is Paula making? How do these reflect her values? A health professional is making judgments about a 'new' patient before he even walks in the door from his notes. How often do you do this? Do you read the notes before seeing a patient for the first time? What may the advantages and disadvantages of this be? Are there certain of your colleagues whose notes you value more than others? Why is this? How do you feel about interacting with a patient who seems to be changing doctors frequently?

Andrew is a personal trainer; he is probably physically fit, maybe muscular, possibly obsessed with exercise. But his records suggest a man with unexplained medical symptoms that could be related to a serious illness. However Paula's partners, whom she trusts, obviously do not think so. They have arranged a few tests 'just to be sure', though it is not entirely clear about what (diabetes, thyroid, anaemia – the tests were a mixed bag). Andrew comes into the room and he does look fit – not fat, walking without obvious pain, but perhaps a little strained, a little ill at ease. Has he lost trust in the other doctors? Does he prefer the feminine touch? Has he heard good things about her? Maybe he is feeling better after a week's rest – though athletes often get very twitchy when told not to exercise. If he still has symptoms what should she do next? She doesn't like to over investigate; she prefers to talk to patients.

Can we imagine what Andrew is thinking? This is more risky guess work. He is a man who is used to fitness, prides himself on his running speed, his muscular torso and the way he looks and feels. He is not used to being ill, apart from temporary aches and pains from over doing the weight training. Perhaps he felt he was not being taken seriously by the other doctors, felt as if he were being fobbed off by 'take two aspirin and have a rest, you'll feel much better in a few days'. As a previous low attender, a person who looks after his health (non-smoker, rare drinker) he expects to be listened to and the doctor to respect the fact he knows his own body. He values his health and, in the same way he helps people to enhance their own fitness, he expects his doctor to sort out his problems professionally and without fuss. After all, the doctor is also a trained professional just like himself.

Dr Chang goes back to the beginning, trying to rid herself of any preconceptions about Andrew from his appearance, demeanour or records. She finds this a good strategy when first seeing a patient with a complicated back story that is not well structured in the records. She indicates to Andrew that this is what she will do: please tell me what has been happening to you from the time just before you noticed your first symptoms. Andrew has told his story several times before: to his partner, the other doctors, a colleague at work and he has rehearsed it to himself. He has also Googled his symptoms. The story is now coloured by the reactions to these various narratives and the rather alarming diagnoses he read on the Internet. He uses words, perhaps unconsciously, to emphasise his concern: the 'aching' of the previous consultations is now quite 'bad pain'; the tiredness is extreme lethargy; the pins and needles are described as electric shocks; the chest pain as a heavy weight. He wants the doctor to take notice; he feels like it is a battle to have his worries acknowledged.

Dr Chang lets him talk, asking just a few questions of clarification. Her mind is sifting through patterns as he speaks, trying to make sense of the symptoms and connect them to a recognisable condition. Andrew is obviously concerned and his affect appears anxious. As Paula has not met him before she is unaware of his premorbid personality. She still has confidence in her partners' appraisal of the situation: it is unlikely that Andrew has a significant medical problem, but she reflects on this and reconsiders – unlikely he has a significant physical problem. She is considering a psychological diagnosis, but this is risky. Andrew's obvious anxiety could be due to his symptoms, or his symptoms could be due to his anxiety. At this point, Dr Chang is more concerned about missing a physical illness than a mental health problem.

Now we can plan Dr Chang's next moves. She should of course examine Andrew – his constellation of symptoms, however, merit a fairly thorough examination and the consultation has already taken 7 minutes. Her professional values would make her feel uncomfortable if she only did a cursory examination or she asked Andrew to come back for another consultation in which to be examined. After all, he has been examined already (though probably not as thoroughly as she would like and not by herself). She needs to make some space in her day. She hates keeping her other patients waiting – this makes her stressed and more likely to interact with patients below her high standards. She decides to ask Andrew to have an ECG (because of the chest pain), which the practice nurse could do at some point that morning, and while Andrew is waiting and then having it done, she can see her next few patients. Basing her decision also on her experience that most patients think that chest pain relates to their hearts, she considers that Andrew's having an ECG might alleviate some of his concerns. She realises however that this is a displacement activity, as the pain does not sound cardiac.

> **Reflection point**
>
> What do you think about this plan? What would you have done differently and why? Is this a valid use of the practice nurse's time? And indeed of Andrew's?

Paula informs Andrew that the nurse will do the ECG. Andrew looks surprised. Paula realises she hasn't yet asked Andrew what he thinks might be wrong. She has been too busy with the large number of conflicting symptoms, their location, duration and precipitating factors. Andrew is in fact concerned he has multiple sclerosis (MS) but has not mentioned this to Paula because she hasn't asked him about his worries. He does say however that he does not think the problem is his heart. His father had a heart problem and this is nothing like that.

Deep breath. What should Paula do now?

- Acknowledge the concerns, but still carry on with the ECG – she needs the space, and it is hard to go back on the rationale for this investigation.
- Discard the ECG and explore Andrew's ideas about his symptoms in more depth.

> **Reflection point**
>
> What affects your decision? Do you involve Andrew in this decision? What does your answer say about your values and what you feel Andrew's values may be?

Enter the practice nurse

The practice nurse working today is Anne Joyner. She is having a busy morning. As well as her own booked appointments, she has been asked to take some urgent blood and do a pregnancy test. She is running about 20 minutes late. Anne is feeling tired. She is trying to lose weight and it is 5 hours since her small bowl of cereal that morning. She has felt embarrassed in her profession to be overweight (BMI 29) and has been working on her diet, having lost 3 kg in the last few weeks. The receptionist rings through to say an extra patient has been added to her list. She sees on the computer that this is a man with chest pain. Chest pain always takes priority in terms of patients being seen quickly and she calls Andrew in within 10 minutes. As he takes off his shirt, she asks him about the chest pain – how long he has had it. Andrew replies that he had chest pain a few days ago but does not have any pain at present. Anne has noticed he is only 29; Andrew has noticed this new health professional is obese.

Reflection point

Consider the issues arising at this point. There are a number of interactions and value systems at play here, including the relationship between Paula and Anne. Do you ever ponder what your patients are thinking about you? Their first impressions?

Andrew thinks: Why am I having an ECG? Now I've mentioned it, I really do want to discuss the possibility of MS. How can a health professional be overweight? I don't have much confidence in her. She's asking me the same questions as the doctor. Don't they read each other's notes? This is a waste of time. Am I seeing the doctor again? I am now getting annoyed. I am going to demand an MRI scan rather than waiting to be offered one.

Anne thinks: Why am I squeezing in this man's ECG? He hasn't got chest pain. He isn't having an MI. It could have waited. I am really hungry and need a break. Look at the way he is looking at me. He obviously thinks I am wasting his time. Paula should have given me more information. And look, the ECG is being reported as normal. I am really not valued here.

Reflection point

So now we have three unhappy and stressed people. Where did it all start to go wrong? What might be the ramifications for Paula and Anne's team working relationships? How might these have been better handled?

One of this practice's values (and probably for most within primary care) is that people with chest pain are a high priority, given that the symptom may signify a serious underlying heart condition such as an acute myocardial infarction (MI). Prompt attention to treatment of MI may help save a life. Obviously a triage process helps in prioritisation by the appropriate health professional weighing up the likelihood that this particular patient with chest pain needs urgent investigation and/or treatment, plus an emergency ambulance for transport to the nearest emergency department. In this particular scenario it is the doctor who first assesses Andrew and it is she who should pass on the relevant information to Anne so that Anne is aware of the seriousness or otherwise of the problem. We can see the common theme again emerge: adequate and timely communication is key. Consider what message Paula should have given to Anne.

However, perhaps there is an alternative viewpoint here. If Paula had played down the possibility of cardiac pathology, Anne might have decided that Andrew could have waited longer for the ECG he does not think he needs. The wait might have reinforced this belief: 'I am obviously not a priority. No-one is taking me seriously and I still haven't had the chance to talk about my concerns'.

Anne is feeling grumpy but her personal and professional values are so ingrained that she cannot just send Andrew back into the waiting room until Paula has another gap in her list to review him. (She presumes that Paula will want to see him with the ECG tracing, though this was not made clear earlier.) Andrew isn't sure what should happen next. He also presumes that he needs to see the GP again in order to carry on the conversation about his condition. What role does Anne have in this narrative of his health? Anne asks him to take a seat and explains that the ECG 'as read by the machine' is normal but that Dr Chang will need to confirm this. Anne's long experience suggests that Andrew is likely to be worried if he has chest pain and no cause is found as yet – though also relieved as this point to be told his test is 'normal' (whatever he thinks that might mean).

'Andrew, do you have any questions before you see Dr Chang again? You might have to wait while she sees more patients.'

Andrew considers whether he wants to involve yet another person is his saga, but he is running out of patience and this invitation is too good to miss. Why not unload his concerns onto this nurse and see what she does about it. His stereotyping of professional values suggests that nurses are caring whereas doctors are efficient. And this less than perfect overweight nurse now seems very human.

'These aches and numbness, and headaches – could it be MS?'

The decision to investigate

Paula and Anne are a team. Their communication processes are variable and in a busy morning's surgery messages are usually passed on via the computer records. Each has to decide whether this is appropriate for each case they deal with. Written messages often miss the nuances of oral communication: the underlying emotions and urgencies that we convey with intonation and rhythm. Written notes are also permanent records of interactions and should require careful thought. They also have the potential to be missed – not read completely as one professional hands over patient care to another. Anne records her consultation in the notes for Paula to read but she wonders if she should also have a word with Paula before Andrew is reviewed. However if Anne disturbs Paula with Andrew's concerns, how will Paula react?

These professional interactions occur regularly through the working day. People who work together frequently begin to read each other's moods and make allowances for good and bad days. However the priority in decisions about what to communicate, when and how, must be based on patient need. In the situation where the doctor and nurse are working in parallel how do they decide together on the best management for the patient and avoid giving mixed or confusing messages and advice?

'These aches and numbness, and headaches – could it be MS?'

Perhaps at this point you are thinking, if only someone had asked Andrew earlier what he thought might be wrong. Well yes – this is part of the ideas, concerns and expectations (ICE) inquiry of the patient-centred approach. However we forget sometimes that patients' concerns are not necessarily static and that they are not always ready to voice them at a particular time. Asking ICE by rote without looking as if you are interested in the answer is unlikely to lead to a frank disclosure. Patients also choose, consciously or unconsciously, who they want to confide in. It might be the professional's manner on the day, or just because the time is right for disclosure. We know that medical and nursing students can pick up patient concerns because they have time to elicit a really full history, and if they do this with feeling and because they are not seen as powerful and threatening, patients confide in them. Some patients are in awe of doctors or particular doctors, preferring the caring manner of the nurse. Anne is in the right place at the right time for Andrew. Paula might feel aggrieved that she did not pick up the cues, that Andrew did not confide in her, that she did not ask the right questions – or she might realise the value of her professional colleague in the team and feel happy that she is now able to continue with the consultation with Andrew's agenda in the open.

The subsequent consultation

Paula reviews Andrew after a short wait. Anne has managed to see her face to face in between patients with the consequence that both of them are now running substantially behind time. The quality of this sort of interaction depends a lot on the amount of respect each professional has for, and shows to, each other. Paula and Anne value each other's professional knowledge and clinical attributes. They don't have the same opinions about everything and, if we explored them in depth, we would find differences in values and approach. Anne advised Paula that Andrew has mentioned he is concerned about having MS but that she has not explored this in any depth, as she knew that Paula would be following him up about the ECG. Anne makes sure she conveys no sense of her frustration at being asked to do the ECG and merely says that she asked Andrew if he had any questions which precipitated his disclosure about MS.

Reflection point

Put yourself now in Paula's shoes. Do you think this is easier to do if you are also a doctor? Why might this be the case? What might you be thinking at this point?

Paula may think:

- Why did Anne pick this up and not me?
- What does Andrew think of me?
- How could I have picked this up?
- Could he have MS?
- Of course he doesn't have MS.
- Do I need to exclude MS?
- Why does he think he may have MS?
- How can I convince him he doesn't have MS?
- I am so far behind.
- How would I diagnose or exclude MS?
- Does he need an MRI?
- Does he merit an MRI?
- It would be a lot quicker if I just filled in the form and gave it to him and had this conversation when he came back with a negative report.
- Unless he does have MS.
- Which he doesn't.

All these thoughts are flashing through Paula's mind as Andrew re-enters the room. After talking to Andrew, Paula has conflicting values. She is fairly sure he doesn't have MS, though the condition is difficult to diagnose. She also realises from the previous consultations and the events of the day so far that Andrew is unlikely to be convinced he doesn't have the condition on her opinion alone. She is in the gatekeeper role of power – she has to make a decision whether to order an expensive investigation and give Andrew some temporary peace of mind as someone is taking him seriously and something is being done, or tell him that in her opinion he doesn't need such an investigation. Her value of being patient-centred is at odds with her feeling of duty to the NHS and proper use of scarce resources. In the end she decides that the MRI might save hassle and time in the long term, but will a negative result really prove to Andrew that he is ok?

A short interlude

Paula and Anne both finish their morning sessions over 40 minutes later than planned. Anne is wondering what the outcome was for Andrew. She could look at Paula's notes on the computer or find Paula to ask. Members of a health care team communicate through patients' records so accessing Andrew's notes is perfectly acceptable as they are both involved in his care. But a few words and an entry for an MRI referral give no indication as to Paula's thought processes. How often do colleagues debrief at the end of a busy morning? A debrief session may be low on the agenda but may be very useful for discussing patients, second opinions, airing grievances and just teambuilding. The more official and timetabled practice meeting might only happen once a week. As people are often so busy the end of clinic coffee time is often a thing of the past. Health professionals finish their appointments at different times and then have administration and other things to do. When one person is free between patients, another may be mid-consultation so discussions are less frequently face-to-face.

A few weeks later

Andrew returns for the result of the MRI scan. Paula first asks him how he is; he says there has been no change in the symptoms and he has been feeling increasingly low. Paula says that the MRI was completely normal, and as she had explained last time, this is a fairly good indication that he does not have MS. Paula knows from her experience that Andrew might react to this news in several ways: he might be extremely relieved that his worst fear has not been realised; he might in some strange way be disappointed that he doesn't have an answer to his problem; he might now worry about something else; he could be more frustrated than ever at the lack of a diagnosis.

The experienced practitioner

While we might employ evidence-based practice for decisions about management, diagnostic acumen through a clinical reasoning process still relies heavily on experience and intuition. Paula knows that unexplained and diverse symptoms can be a sign of depression (there is plenty of evidence for this) and she is picking up cues from Andrew that there are parts of his story he hasn't yet divulged (her intuition).

An aside – Author's personal note: I have to exercise some caution here. As a young GP I was encouraged to read 'The Doctor, His Patient and the Illness' by Michael Balint (1957), which focuses on understanding the emotional content of patient-GP consultations. I remember clearly the idea of the 'Balint flash': the doctor has a sudden flash of understanding that illuminates his or her relationship with the patient. This could happen after many consultations in which there might appear to be some underlying blockage to a successful outcome or an agreed management plan. The patient would say something and – FLASH – all was revealed. The doctor would realise that his/her own low mood was mirroring the previously unrecognised depression of the patient. The doctor would then make an empathic statement, 'I can see you are really quite unhappy', and the patient would reveal all (and be cured). Though I do admit this is a very simplistic view of a complex process: this is my fantasy about the flash, and it very rarely happened. I am now considering whether Paula should have a flash and Andrew's underlying mental health problems will surface.

Andrew's story is based loosely on a real patient, interwoven with other consultation experiences to ensure he cannot be identified. The rest of his story did take a few consultations but for the purposes of this chapter, there is a flash, and Andrew talks about his traumatic experience. Many patients presenting in this way will not have such past histories. And some with these symptoms will have MS or another underlying physical condition.

The experienced practitioner continued

Andrew recounts that when he was 18 he found his mother dead at home – she had cut her wrists and taken an overdose. He had had some counselling at the time but 'wasn't the type' to talk about his problems. He had thrown himself into physical fitness and personal training, and found that excessive exercise was a way to keep his mind off things until just recently. He got engaged about 6 months ago and is thinking how sad it will be that his mother won't be at his wedding. His symptoms started soon after his engagement and his concerns about MS were precipitated by Googling 'strange feelings in arms'. Paula diagnoses post-traumatic stress disorder (PTSD) and anxiety.

Medically unexplained symptoms (MUS)

Unexplained symptoms are frustrating and dissatisfying for both patient (Jackson & Kroenke, 2001) and clinician (Hahn, 2001). This frustration can lead to referral of a patient along the health professional chain via the primary care team (for example, practice nurse to nurse practitioner to GP) and onto secondary care. Uncertainty regarding diagnosis is also one factor that influences doctors (Bradley, 1992), and no doubt nurse practitioners, to prescribe: treating symptoms rather than underlying causes.

Symptoms that cannot be adequately diagnosed as being due to organic illness are referred to as medically unexplained symptoms (Reid et al., 2001) or MUS. If an organic disease is present, the symptoms are not consistent with that disease or are out of proportion to it (Smith et al., 2006). When the symptoms are severe enough to impact on a person's ability to work, perform routine daily tasks or fulfil social responsibilities, the condition is referred to as somatisation disorder. Patients with MUS account for about one fifth of general practice consultations (De Waal et al., 2004), while about 4% of the general population have more complex and chronic multiple functional symptoms, most of them women: an average of 10–15 per GP (Bass & May, 2002). Patients are often referred for a specialist opinion; in fact about one third of new referrals to medical out-patients are people with MUS (Reid et al., 2003). While MUS is not a diagnosis as such, the label is often one of exclusion, i.e. once other possible conditions have been ruled out by a careful history, physical examination and relevant investigations. Neither patient nor doctor wants to miss a serious underlying disease. The most common eventual underlying diagnoses are anxiety, depression and/or panic disorders (Burton et al., 2011). However because the predictive value of unexplained symptoms for anxiety and depression is low, GPs are not justified in screening patients presenting with MUS for these conditions (van Boven et al., 2011).

Other diagnoses relating to MUS, which focus on the symptomatology, have been proposed (Box 6.1); these are included in the Diagnostic and Statistical Manual of Mental Disorders (DSM-IV), published by the American Psychiatric Association (APA, 1999). The

DSM-IV is one of the major classification systems for mental health problems. It has a multi-dimensional or multiaxial approach to diagnosis, acknowledging that social and other factors do impact on patients' mental health (Box 6.2).

Box 6.1: Diagnoses for MUS (medically unexplained symptoms) (Adapted from Stone, 2011)

- Based on symptom count: somatisation disorder (Axis I)
    Chronic and severe condition with minimum of eight symptoms beginning before age 30.
- Functional somatic disorders (Axis III):
    Includes irritable bowel syndrome and fibromyalgia.
- Incorporating cognitive, behavioural and affective elements.
    Hypochondriasis (Axis I):
        Fear of having a serious disease lasting at least 6 months despite appropriate investigationand reassurance.
    Complex somatic symptom disorder (proposed for Axis I):
        One or more somatic symptoms, includes high level of health-related anxiety, excessive time and energy spent on symptoms or concerns.

Box 6.2: Multi-axial approach to psychiatric diagnosis from DSM-IV

Axis I: Clinical syndromes
- The clinical diagnoses, e.g. anxiety, depression, bipolar disorder.

Axis II: Developmental disorders and personality disorders
- Developmental disorders are those which typically become evidence in childhood such as autism and learning disabilities.
- Personality disorders are clinical syndromes that affect a person's interaction with society. Examples are borderline personality disorder, antisocial personality disorder.

Axis III: Physical conditions
- These conditions affect the development, continuance or exacerbation of disorders from axes I and II. Examples are head injury and multi-infarct dementia.

Axis IV: Severity of psychosocial and environmental stressors
- Life events such as bereavement, house move, becoming unemployed etc which affect the mental condition.

Making a diagnosis of mental illness after exclusion of physical disease is not ideal. Yet health professionals may be more concerned about missing cancer or a treatable condition than depression or anxiety. By the time the practitioner broaches the possibility of a mental health problem, the patient might have had many investigations and a long list of differential diagnoses. This pattern is not helped by the specialisation of much of secondary care. Patients are referred from the gastroenterologist to the neurologist to the cardiologist and so on with a subsequent lack of holistic care. But this searching for a diagnosis is reinforced by our own experiences of patients who eventually are shown to have MS, or coeliac disease or ovarian cancer. We all know of people, and our patients read their stories in the media, who were labelled neurotic or depressed or personality disorder, and who subsequently died of unrecognised pathology. In terms of values, it seems better to have a physical illness than a mental one, the latter being associated with stigma and instability.

Patients with MUS are often given unfortunate tags such as frequent attenders, heartsink patients, doctor shoppers and somatisers, saying more about the values of the professional, who uses such labels, than the person who consults. O'Dowd coined the term heartsink in the UK in 1988 (O'Dowd, 1988). A decade earlier an American psychiatrist called Groves talked of 'hateful' patients (Groves, 1978). What this says about their values we can only surmise. Discussions about interactions with these types of patients typically focus on the doctor as they engender many different emotions in the doctor (Thistlethwaite & Morris, 2006). It is difficult to maintain empathy. The frustration of the professional mirrors the frustration of the patient and this can be acknowledged: 'The fact that I haven't been able to help you must be very frustrating'.

How does the patient label the professional? Probably not hateful but possibly uncaring, arrogant, difficult. This may be why they choose another practitioner, a different type of professional, a complementary therapist: in the hope of finding one to listen.

Thinking back to Andrew and Paula: Paula began by eliciting as full a history as possible within her limited consultation time. A framework for such consultations is shown in Box 6.3. Not all these steps can/should be covered in one consultation.

Box 6.3: Stages in the process of 'difficult' consultations – Adapted from Bass & May (2002) and Thistlethwaite & Morris (2006)

Prior to the consultation: review the patient's records including investigations, referrals and treatments with their timeframe

Information gathering

- Gather information about the presenting complaint.
- Elicit the patient's story including social background and life events.
- Use open questions and try not to adopt a biomedical model.
- Gather information about the previous medical history and its timeframe in the patient's own words including treatment and the patient's feeling about this.
- Explore the patient's ideas, concerns, expectations and values.
- Do not assume that the patient wants investigations or a prescription.
- Discuss the patient's experiences with medical services and previous doctors, and find out why he/she has consulted **you** today.
- Reframe the physical symptoms if possible to show links between life events (with caution).
- Remember to reflect on how you are feeling as this may mirror the patient's mood, e.g. frustrated, low.

Information sharing, shared decision making and management

- Formulate a problem list with the patient and priorities for management.
- Discuss the probability that there is no cure but rather an improvement in well-being to some extent and that this will take time.
- Discuss the use of any drugs, prescribed or OTC, and decide which are necessary.
- Check that the patient has understood.
- Encourage patient to take responsibility for health.
- Avoid referral.
- Make informal contract with patient to consult with you only and at predefined intervals.
- Involve family member or friend to help support patient in managing the problems.

Reflection point

Consider a patient you have interacted with who had multiple symptoms like Andrew. How did this make you feel? How do you think your patient felt? Did you refer the patient to another professional or team member for respite from your relationship? What might another health professional add to the skill set? Have you ever referred to a patient as heart sink? Consider the values-based practice issues here in such a term – will you think twice about using such a label again?

Conclusion

We should not think 'difficult patient' but rather 'difficult consultation'. Health professionals are not alone in health care; they do not have to interact with patients as the sole practitioner. The team should be supportive but there needs to be time in a busy day to debrief and discuss difficult consultations with colleagues. Values-based practice and patient-centredness is not just about agreeing to a patient's wants, but exploring values to determine in partnership what the patient's needs may be.

References

APA. (1994). *Diagnostic and statistical manual of mental disorders* (4th edition). Arlington: APA.

Balint M. (1957). *The doctor, his patient and the illness*. London: Pitman Medical.

Bass C and May S. (2002). Chronic multiple functional somatic symptoms. *BMJ*, **325**;323–326.

Bradley CP. (1992). Factors which influence the decision whether or not to prescribe: the dilemma facing general practitioners. *British Journal of General Practice*, **42**; 454–458.

Burton C, McGorm K, Weller D and Sharpe M. (2011). Depression and anxiety in patients repeatedly referred to secondary care with medically unexplained symptoms: a case-control study. *Psychological Medicine*, **41**;555–563.

De Waal MWM, Arnold IA, Eekhof JAH and Van Hemert AM. (2004). Somatoform disorders in general practice: prevalence, functional impairment and co-morbidity with anxiety and depression. *British Journal of Psychology*, **184**;470–476.

Groves JE. (1978). Taking care of the hateful patient. *New England Journal of Medicine*, **298**;317–318.

Hahn SR. (2001). Physical symptoms and physician-experienced difficulty in the physician-patient relationship. *Annals of Internal Medicine*, **134**;897–904.

Jackson AL and Kroenke K. (2001). The effect of unmet expectations among adults presenting with physical symptoms. *Annals of Internal Medicine*, **134**;889–897.

O'Dowd TC. (1988). Five years of heartsink patients in general practice. *BMJ*, **325**;1342–1345.

Reid S, Crayford T, Patel A, Wessely S and Hotopf M. (2003). Frequent attenders in secondary care: a 3-year follow-up study of patients with medically unexplained symptoms. *Psychological Medicine*, **33**;519–524.

Reid S, Wessely S, Crayford T and Hotopf M. (2001). Medically unexplained symptoms in frequent attenders of secondary health care: retrospective cohort study. *BMJ*, **322**;767–771.

Smith RC, Lyles JS, Gardiner JC, et al. (2006). Primary care clinicians treat patients with medically unexplained symptoms: a randomized controlled trial. *Journal of General Internal Medicine*, **21**;671–677.

Stone L. (2011). Explaining the unexplainable. *Australian Family Physician*, **40**;440–444.

Thistlethwaite JE and Morris P. (2006). *The patient-doctor consultation in primary care. Theory and practice*. London: RCGP.

van Boven K, Lucassen P, van Revesteijn H, et al. (2011). Do unexplained symptoms predict anxiety and depression? *British Journal of General Practice*, **61**;387–388.

7

A request for strong analgesia: honesty and trust

This chapter explores another area of difficult patient interactions and the issue of trust. Inappropriate requests are fairly common in primary care, but we need to consider who defines 'appropriate'. Communication between professionals is again a focus.

Maggie Brookner, a nurse practitioner of 5 years experience, is working in a walk-in centre on Saturday evening with GP Dr Paul Mathur. Paul recently passed his membership examination of the Royal College of General Practitioners (giving him the qualification MRCGP) and has been working as a locum in different parts of the country while he decides where to look for a permanent practice.

Maggie's next patient is Moira Whelan. She has not been seen in the centre before. She is a well-dressed and well-spoken 35 year old. She sits down with some difficulty and begins to tell Maggie about the pain in her back. This started the night before while she was bending down to empty her washing machine. She has been in discomfort all night and has just about managed a day's work as a secretary by taking ibuprofen and paracetamol. She asks if she can have 'something stronger for the pain' otherwise she doesn't think she will sleep at all for a second night.

Reflection point

What are your immediate thoughts given this very common scenario? What has prompted these thoughts from your experience, profession and/or training?

You may have thought:

- Back pain is common, sounds like a familiar story.
- I have had back pain and it is painful – she certainly looks like she is having trouble sitting and standing.
- Is this person just out to get some strong analgesics from me?
- Is she credible?
- What if I give her pills and she is an addict or selling them on?
- What if she is genuine and I refuse to help?
- Does she look like an addict?
- Why hasn't she contacted her own GP? She has had all day to do so.
- She probably knows I don't have any medical records for her.
- This is going to take some time to sort out.

> **Reflection point**
> What does your immediate reaction say about your values? If you felt suspicious straight away what does this indicate about you? If you are empathic why might this be the case? How do you think other members of your team would react to this request and why?

Value judgments

This is a very common consultation and the health professional involved needs to make a fairly quick value judgment based on a short history, an examination, no records and intuition. Intuition (the ability to acquire immediate knowledge without the use of reason) is often guided by our values. Some health professionals may never prescribe strong analgesia to patients they haven't met before or have no prior history of. Indeed, your practice may have a policy, guided by the professionals' values and perhaps even indicated in reception, that you only prescribe analgesia/strong painkillers to registered patients.

But this is a walk-in centre and many patients will have genuine pain, following trauma or other conditions that are not serious enough for attendance and management at the Emergency Department, but that require same day prescriptions. Could your policy disadvantage some of the vulnerable members of the community?

Maggie doesn't know Paul very well either. She has a choice of passing Moira over to him for a second opinion. She wonders what he might think of her then – she is proud of her status as a nurse practitioner and likes to practise as autonomously as possible when she can. However she would not prescribe opioids for a patient without discussing the situation with a doctor. First of all, however, she decides she will ask some more questions. She realises that her value judgment is being affected by Moira's quiet demeanour; in fact Moira is very similar to many of her friends. Maggie knows she would be much more suspicious if the patient were younger, scruffy and male.

Certain drugs raise strong emotions

Being asked to prescribe certain types of drugs precipitates diverse emotions in professionals: some of these are values-related, and others professional and intellectual. Patients demonstrating potential drug-seeking behaviour are worrying for the prescriber, who is concerned about being manipulated, while not wanting to appear to be overly suspicious of someone who might have a genuine problem. (And here think of the fact that labelling a problem genuine or false is a value judgment in itself.) These interactions make forming the expected 'therapeutic alliance' very difficult, and the patient–physician relationship is likely to be strained (Finch, 1993).

The dilemma involved in the decision to prescribe or not to prescribe has various consequences such as: being time-consuming, causing inner conflicts, worrying about the patient and doing the right thing, discontent with whatever action is taken and feeling incompetent (Bendtsen et al., 1999). In this scenario there is also the potential to become annoyed with a colleague, who passes the buck or acts inappropriately. When clinicians feel under pressure, and particularly when they need to take time to 'sort out' one patient while others are waiting, they are more likely to make mistakes and lose empathy and judgment.

The battle with some clients to get clinicians to prescribe drugs is often discussed at professional development sessions. The prescriber is in a powerful position in relation to the prescription pad. Success is often seen as not prescribing when patients ask (or we may say demand if making a value judgment). This demand is often for antibiotics, analgesics and sleeping pills. Do you recognise any of the remarks in Box 7.1?

Box 7.1: What we might be thinking or saying

- She wanted amoxicillin but I wouldn't give it to her.
- It's only a sore throat.
- He can't be in that much pain, he still manages to get to the pub.
- Why do they still expect antibiotics for sore throats?
- I don't believe he lost his prescription.
- How could she have come on holiday without her co-codamol?
- He's obviously up-to-something – he's unemployed and has lots of tattoos.

Different values – different people

One of the attributes commonly considered a key feature of health professionals is altruism, which may be defined as an unselfish concern for the welfare of others. Health professionals on the whole put the needs of patients before themselves, though the extent of this may vary. Health professionals are increasingly being trained to be empathic; they also feel uncomfortable when they start to mistrust a patient: is this patient telling the truth? Eliciting histories is a skill based on the premise that most of the time the patient is telling the truth, though they may forget certain aspects of their past or interpret things in a certain light depending on their values and health beliefs. However the majority of patients do not deliberately set out to falsify their stories or tell lies. So how much should a health professional believe? Is there ever an excuse for confronting a patient and accusing him or her of not telling the truth (which sounds better than accusing him or her of lying)? The question also arises as to who defines the needs of patients. The hallmark of paternalism and doctor-centred care, for example, is that the clinician decides on what the patient needs, and contrasts this with what the patient wants.

In terms of pain relief, the patient needs a respite from pain and there are a number of good analgesics that can provide this. The patient, however, may want a stronger painkiller than the doctor is prepared to prescribe, for a number of reasons:

- The patient feels that paracetamol and other over the counter (OTC) preparations are only for minor aches and pains and that they will not be effective against more acute and less frequent pains such as backache.
- There is no point in coming to the clinic to get an OTC tablet unless it is free – and many doctors now will not write prescriptions for OTC drugs to discourage patients from attending for minor problems; so if someone decides to attend the surgery rather than the pharmacy, they want a prescription drug.
- The patient has tried other drugs and they either do not provide relief for long enough or they have side effects such as indigestion.
- Paracetamol is dangerous – you can only buy a few at a time which is proof of this.
- Stronger painkillers make you feel nice as well as pain free.
- The patient is addicted to the feeling of the drugs.

The doctor (or nurse practitioner) may not be prepared to prescribe also for various reasons:

- The prescriber is responsible for the prescription if the patient is adversely affected by the drugs and the prescriber has not taken reasonable precautions in eliciting and checking the history.
- There is a feeling that the patient is manipulating the prescriber's emotions, playing on the sense of altruism, to gain something over and above necessary medical care.
- The patient appears untrustworthy – this will depend on the prescriber's previous experiences and values in relation to age, clothing, apparent intelligence, whether employed etc.
- The prescriber does not believe that the pain is so severe it will not settle with simple analgesia – here there is a lot of decision making based on the way the patient acts: how does a patient act out their pain?

This is an interesting point – how do we represent and describe pain? We expect people with back pain to have problems doing certain movements, for example we watch them closely when climbing up onto and off the examination couch, when they sit, stand and walk. We look for facial grimaces. For other pains we watch for flinching when touched, or even tears coming to the eyes. But we know that people have different thresholds for pain. We can attempt a more 'scientific' measure: what is your pain like on a scale of 1 to 10 if 1 is no pain and 10 is the worst pain you can think of? But this presupposes that the patient has a scale similar to ours (his 8 is our 8 and a fairly objective measure) or that his scale reflects a more subjective measure at this point in time – well this is the most severe pain I have ever had up till now, but I haven't had a heart attack or given birth. The pain scale is useful for measuring change in awareness of pain, but we are unlikely to make a decision totally about prescribing based on a score of 9 in a person who looks comfortable but is asking for strong opioids. For of course patients can learn to play this game.

If we say someone has a low threshold for pain – is that a value judgment? Do we expect people to pull themselves together and get on with it? Do we base that expectation on how we ourselves cope with pain? I never take painkillers – I prefer to let nature take its course. I try to take two paracetamol as soon as I feel a headache coming on, that way it never gets too bad. If my knee is playing up I take a day off work. If my back is bad I go to the gym to get it moving.

Now do we think that Maggie and Paul might approach this patient in different ways? Is this likely to be due to their profession, their personal experiences, their professional experiences, their training? In terms of stereotypes, considering that Maggie is a nurse and 'caring', her nursing values may suggest trusting the patient and prescribing; whereas Paul as a doctor may be seen as more 'clinical' and even discerning, and he may decide not to trust the patient and therefore not prescribe. Of course our stereotyping of the professions in this way in itself reflects our values.

Maggie might decide to refer Moira onto Paul; Paul may feel aggrieved about this and that might affect his consultation, or he might feel that this reflects the nature of the health professional hierarchy – the doctor is better at dealing with these sticky problems.

Community values

Beyond the immediate health care team we also need to think about the community's values in terms of drugs of addiction. Here we have an immediate problem in defining who the community is. There are obviously laws about how prescription only drugs may be prescribed, dispensed and disposed of. And there are legal ramifications for ignoring or flouting these rules. However, as we have noted before, our values may be at odds with the law. For example health professionals with access to drugs through their work may take a strong analgesic that was not prescribed for them and cannot be obtained OTC.

Reflection point

Think of situations this may occur: which are you ok with? Which are officially illegal, or unprofessional? Have you taken any medication, or given medication to a family member, for a condition that you would not have prescribed for a patient?

In the following scenario you have troubling back pain, which you want to treat so you can continue to work at your clinic. Paracetamol has not worked. Do you:

- Take a drug prescribed for a family member or friend?
- Take a drug that a patient has returned to you because of side effects?
- Take a drug from the drug cupboard at work, which contains samples?
- Make an appointment with your GP for advice and a possible prescription?
- Ring your GP and ask for a prescription?

You may think any of the top three are OK – you are doing this in a spirit of altruism: you need to work to avoid putting extra pressure on your colleagues. Now, what if you start to do this on a regular basis? Leaving aside the issue of pain that should be investigated by someone rather than relying on self-diagnosis, at what point does your behaviour step over a boundary? Some might say the first time you took a tablet, others when this became a habit. Now you could apply a test of what would your peers think? The other members of the team? The pharmacist? Your GP? Your patients? Your professional registration body? All of these could be defined as members of the community.

But within the community there are also the drug seekers and addicts who may have a different set of values in terms of taking analgesics and obtaining drugs. Many people who are addicted to prescription drugs originally obtained their prescription in good faith and, for some reason, continued to receive repeat prescriptions without adequate follow-up or discussion. They then meet a health professional who wants to reduce their dose, wean them off their addiction and treat them with something very different like physiotherapy or cognitive behavioural therapy. Whose 'fault' is the addiction?

Addiction raises mixed emotions in professionals: to some it is a lifestyle problem that can be managed with will power and motivation; to others a physical and mental health problem that requires professional help. Does one's viewpoint on this depend on the addiction? People may be addicted to heroin, cigarettes, gambling, benzodiazepines, food, sex. Some of these are more physical than psychological – some habits more than addiction.

What could happen in the consultation?

Maggie has been processing her possible courses of action while listening to Moira telling her story. She knows that patients seeking drugs can be manipulative and plausible; she also realises that she wants to believe Moira and trust her because she would hate to leave someone in genuine pain all night. She postpones her decision while asking more questions about the pain. There is nothing to prove or disprove the necessity for analgesia or the possibility that this story has been told several times before. She could ask Moira for her GP's number and ring to find out more about her, but this will take time and the practice might not be open at this hour in the evening.

Maggie knows that there are two fallback positions:

- Invoke the practice policy of not recommending anything stronger than OTC medication for new or unknown patients without records.
- Asking Paul for an opinion.

She is able to go against the policy if she can justify her actions but doesn't feel confident on this occasion. She decides to get the second opinion. What should she say to Moira (Box 7.2)? The last option reflects what Moira is really thinking – but would you say this?

Box 7.2: What would you say to Moira?

- I would like the doctor to give a second opinion about your back pain to rule out anything more serious than a muscular problem.
- Only the doctor can prescribe the type of medication you want.
- To be honest, and as I am sure you are aware of the problem, certain people come into the clinic looking for painkillers for themselves or others because they are addicted or are selling on the pills. I want to trust you but am not entirely sure therefore I would like the doctor to see you.

Honesty is a value

How honest should we be with patients? Probably most professionals would not advocate outright lying to patients or other staff, but you may consider a 'white lie' perfectly acceptable. If we think of a white lie as bending the truth, this may also be alright depending on the context. With the options above, the first two may be true, but are they honest? They are not really the reason why Maggie has decided to act the way she has. Is honesty the best policy? Is honesty a practice value?

Other examples of 'honest' statements are:

- I don't know what is wrong with you but I will try to find out.
- I don't think there is anything physically wrong with you at all.
- I think you are just trying to have a few days off work.
- I am sure you are trying to defraud your insurance company.
- I can't remember the name of the drug I want to prescribe, so I am going to Google it.
- I don't know who you are and therefore can't remember what your problem is.
- You really do make my heart sink and I would prefer it if you saw one of the other nurses next time.

There is a difference between being honest in terms of what you think (or conjecture, or are suspicious of) and being honest in terms of hard facts. The first is a subjective opinion while the latter is undeniable. As has happened on several occasions I have examined patients and found physical signs highly suggestive of cancer. If the patient wasn't expecting this (the patient's elicited ideas focusing on other conditions), should you say 'I think you might have cancer' if there is any possibility it might be something else, and the patient doesn't ask specifically what the diagnosis might be? So I examine a patient with rectal bleeding who has a rectal mass – very likely cancer but I suggest piles and a referral. We might be

> **Box 7.3:** From my experience
>
> Once a patient I knew fairly well brought her 7 month old infant into see me. The boy had unexplained bruises around his eyes. I was sure that there was a very low probability of child abuse, but there had to be a reason for the physical signs. I told the mother I had to send the child to hospital and that the staff there would have to rule out non-accidental injury. I also said that while I did not think this was a likely possibility, I had to consider this as a potential diagnosis. She said she was grateful for my honesty. I thought later about the motive for that honesty – was it helping me more than her? I did not want to write anything in the admission letter that I would not say to her face and she needed to be prepared for questions when she and her son arrived on the ward. In the event the child was found to have a malignancy and I was involved in his care for many more years. Would I have been as honest if I thought that NAI was very likely in case the mother did not go to the hospital?

asked: what do you think it is doctor? Then we have to make a split second decision how to answer. Patients may see us hesitate, and depending on the circumstances, may fear the worst. Unless you are a good actor, it can be difficult to lie and not be caught out. We can avoid a direct response. For example to a woman with a breast lump we can say 'don't worry' when we suggest referring her to the specialist, or even worse 'there's nothing to worry about, you're going to be alright'.

We no doubt value honesty in our record keeping. Have you ever forgotten a patient's BP reading by the time you are recording it and therefore have written down what you think it was?

If as professionals we value honesty, we probably also expect our patients and other members of the team to be honest. While we may be suspicious of patients asking for analgesics, as in this case, we usually believe what people tell us when we are eliciting a history. However we do know that patients forget their medical histories, that they remember them inaccurately, that they leave things out to look better or because they think certain symptoms are trivial, that they might not admit to illegal behaviour. How often do patients actually lie though? Does telling a nurse you smoke 5 a day when in fact you smoke 15 count as a lie or bending the truth? Why does a patient lie like this? What does it say about their expectations and values?

Consider why a patient might bend the truth about smoking, alcohol consumption, illicit drug use or diet (Box 7.4). All these reasons show something about a person's relationship with a health professional. They may interact differently if asked by a nurse rather than by a doctor, or in hospital rather than in the community: is this about perceptions of authority or power? While patients probably understand something about confidentiality, they may consider that it is not wise to admit to illegal activity, and moreover do not want anything recorded about such behaviour.

The truth, the whole truth?

Can you tell when a person is lying? There may be something in the body language, but it can be subtle, and some people are just very good at telling lies. So there is no absolutely sure way of detecting liars and no consensus amongst experts about the better methods. Cultural background may affect non-verbal cues for example. Shifting gaze, thinking too long about an answer to a simple question, fidgeting, are possible pointers. Confronting a patient and accusing them of lying is not recommended. Asking 'are you sure' might also sound as if you

Box 7.4: Reasons to bend the truth

- They feel ashamed about their habit.
- They promised they would stop/reduce and are too embarrassed to admit failure – they want to save face.
- They don't want another lecture.
- They lie to their family and friends and so it is a habit.
- They think we may judge them.
- They want to be praised/liked.
- They are afraid we may withhold treatment if they continue to abuse their bodies.
- They don't really keep count and guess at a figure.
- They don't want to get into trouble with the police.
- They don't think it is any of the professional's business.
- They really don't note what they are eating.
- They don't think that crisps count as food.

don't trust them. You could say: many people underestimate how much they drink. Do you think you might have more than that a day/week?

Reflection point

What do you do if a patient accuses you of lying? It would depend if you were! You can reflect the question back – what makes you ask that? It is more likely that you will be asked; is that true? Is there anything you are not telling me?

Blood and urine tests may indicate that there is a lack of honesty on the patient's part in relation to drug taking. There is of course formal testing of drug addicts when they are being treated. Rather than continue to increase and add anti-hypertensive medication to a patient's regimen whose blood pressure is not falling, ask if they are taking the tablets as advised. A person may not volunteer non-adherence, but may admit this when directly asked.

Trust and its importance in interactions

Trust is obviously linked to values of honesty and integrity (Lafolette, 1993): we do not trust people we believe are lying. However as trust implies vulnerability on the part of the person who trusts, as professionals we are unlikely to talk about trusting patients with the same meaning as patients' stating that they trust their professionals. Patients trust their professionals to do the right thing and to get it right. If Moira does genuinely have back pain and has no other motive to ask for analgesia than pain relief, she attends the surgery trusting that the health professional she consults will treat her appropriately. She might feel vulnerable to being mistrusted (she may realise that there are problems with people seeking drugs inappropriately). If trust breaks down, patients may not adhere to medication regimens, may seek other forms of help or make a complaint.

MORI (Market and Opinion Research International) regularly polls the British public to ascertain the level of trust in professions, including doctors, teachers, judges, politicians and journalists. Consistently in the last 30 years, doctors have topped the trust league table; teachers and clergy are just behind them (Royal College of Physicians, 2009). However, MORI also points out that factors such as gender, age, employment status, social class and ethnicity all influence trust. Social class differences are apparent in levels of trust for nearly all the professions. Those belonging to less affluent backgrounds (social classes DE) are generally less likely to trust professionals than those belonging to social classes AB (Royal College of Physicians 2009).

Health professionals generally trust one another, otherwise they would find it difficult to refer to each other and/or work together in other ways. But consider, if you are able to say you don't trust a certain doctor or other health professional, why is that? And if that person has lost your trust, is he or she a risk to patients or underperforming in some other way? If you can say 'I would never refer a patient to Mr X at the local hospital', should something be done about Mr X and what?

Moira and Paul have not worked together for long but they trust each other on the basis that they are health professionals and employed in the same practice. 'She wouldn't be working here if she wasn't ok; he wouldn't have qualified unless he was fit to practise.' Personal trust takes longer; we need to work with someone for a while to know what they are skilled at, what they are capable of and what their scope of practice is, etc. As we noted in Chapter 2, Box 2.5, absence of trust leads to team dysfunction. Some of the symptoms are that team members conceal their weaknesses and mistakes from one another, they hesitate to ask for or offer help, they jump to conclusions about each other's actions (and values), they fail to recognise each other's skills and they often hold grudges (Lencioni, 2002).

Intuition and risk assessment

Patients who are drug seekers may be desperate and potentially violent. Perhaps perceptions, or value judgments such as this, make health professionals wary of certain types of consultations. How often does a patient become angry if we refuse to give them the medication they are requesting (or demanding)? When might such anger manifest as verbal or even physical violence?

Health care settings usually have a zero policy to violent or abusive behaviour, but this policy only kicks in after the event in terms of removal of such patients. Health professionals, unsurprisingly, value their safety and do not want to be in fear of abuse at work. How does a health professional assess potential risk? Again, value judgments based on experience, own gender and a number of other factors come into play, such as personal biases. There is probably no systematic weighing of these factors but rather instinct or intuition (Magin et al., 2008), which of course may be misguided. We possibly may also take into consideration the circumstances and are likely to feel more vulnerable when the surgery is less busy, all the remaining staff are female and it is dark outside.

Consider Moira requesting analgesia, and how she might be feeling. Scenario 1: Moira is genuinely in pain and has been very honest and open. She trusts the health professional to listen to her and, while knowing that some people do seek drugs, she is sure that Maggie is sympathetic and able to discern her honesty. She is glad she is seeing a female and a nurse as she assumes a certain amount of caring. Moira does feel intimidated by male professionals especially if they challenge her story and is more likely not to press her case if consulting a male doctor. Scenario 2: Moira has some pain but is taking regular analgesia over and above the recommended dose. She usually gets her prescription from her registered practice and the amount she receives is controlled through a contract she has made with her regular GP. However every so often she attends a walk-in centre to get more when she is running low before her next scheduled consultation. She assumes her doctor is sent a record of this but he has never mentioned it. One time she did give the wrong practice address when asked by the receptionist and again this was not challenged. She is surprised how trusting people seem to be and she is counting on this. She tries to see a female practitioner, as again they seem more empathic though even then they will only prescribe a few tablets to 'tide her over until she sees her regular doctor'. Scenario 3: This is the third walk-in centre Moira has attended this month. She gives her real name and address as written on her driving licence but gives different addresses for her GP. She does have some back pain but both she and her partner are addicted to codeine. She obtains a prescription about 50% of the time. She prefers female professionals, nurses or younger doctors. She rather enjoys the role-play but if the drugs are refused she does not get angry but leaves so that there is no chance the police are called.

Conclusion

Health professionals are probably naturally trusting and appear trustworthy to their patients. Trust may be lost and certainly this is likely if one or other of the partnership lie. White lies may fit with a professional's value of not hurting a patient through the unadorned truth, but the professional is then making a judgment with which neither her colleagues nor her patient agrees.

References

Bendtsen P, Hensing G, Ebeling C and Pain AS. (1999). What are the qualities of dilemmas experienced when prescribing opioids in general practice? *Pain*, **82**;89–96.

Finch J. (1993). Prescription drug abuse. *Primary Care*, **20**; 231–239.

Lafollette, H. (1993). Personal Relationships. In: Singer P (Ed). *A companion to ethics*. Oxford: Blackwell. p331.

Lencioni P. (2002). *The five dysfunctions of a team*. Lafayette: The Table Group.

Magin P, Adams J, Joy E, Ireland M, Heaney S and Darab S. (2008). General practitioners' assessment of risk of violence in their practice: Results from a qualitative study. *Journal of Evaluation in Clinical Practice*, **14**;385–390.

Royal College of Physicians. (2009). Available at: http://www.rcplondon.ac.uk/media/Press-releases/Documents/RCP-Trust-in-Professions-2009-summary.pdf (Accessed December 2011).

8 Asylum seekers and refugees: working across cultures

In this chapter we look at values relating to culture: working with people from other cultures (professionals and patients) and problems with bias and racism. These are difficult conversations and require us to reflect on our practice, how we relate to others from different backgrounds and with different languages from our own. The difference may be related to upbringing, social class and education as well as ethnicity, country of origin and customs.

Soraya and her son

Stonybrook Health Centre is a large multiprofessional health care provider in the inner city area of a deprived city. A high proportion of its patients do not speak English as a first, or even second language. The local population is multiethnic, multicultural and comes from more than 40 countries.

> **Reflection point**
>
> What difficulties do you envisage (or have) working and/or living in a place like Stonybrook? What might be the advantages as well as disadvantages? What, if any changes, might health professionals need to make in order to provide the optimal service for their clientele?

One morning Soraya Nimbini, accompanied by her 7 year old son Sukesh, attends the surgery. She was seen by one of the GPs as a new patient last week and in accordance with practice policy she was given an appointment with nurse practitioner Gina Caruso for a new patient check today. Gina is mentoring a fourth year medical student Philip Rohde during the morning. Soraya arrives 15 minutes late. She holds a tattered document in Arabic and simple English outlining her story of abuse at the hands of various militia in East Africa. Philip says hello but she ignores him and asks Gina to read it. The GP's notes state that she is an asylum seeker, currently living with her husband and his older sister; the latter has a work visa for the UK. The GP also wrote that Soraya is trying to get pregnant but has not been able to do so for the last 6 months. Soraya's English is difficult to understand and she appears to be very shy. In particular, she does not look at Philip when he asks her questions. She is wearing a head scarf and abaya (full length garment covering the whole body including the arms) but does not have her face covered. The appointment is for herself but she also wants Sukesh to be checked over.

Reflection point

What feelings do you have on reading the scenario and why? Do these say anything about your values? What might Soraya's values be?

At the end of the consultation, which took 30 minutes, Gina asks Philip for comments on the content and process of the interaction, what he thinks went well and what could have been done differently. He replies: I found this consultation really frustrating, as I didn't think we could really understand what the patient wanted. I felt awkward because she obviously didn't want to interact with me, but you did ask her if it was all right if I stayed. It is very difficult trying to be patient-centred, as we are taught, when the patient's English is not so good and they can't express their ideas and concerns, even though I would imagine this lady has many anxieties and health issues. The fact she was late meant that other people ended up waiting longer than their appointment times, but I liked the way you didn't try to hurry her, though such a long appointment must mean that other patients don't get their full time – or else everyone has to work later. I feel helpless in the face of traumatic patient experiences; I am sure the letter only touched on part of what she must have been through, though I suppose, according to the media, that some people do forge their documents in order to get housed here. I suppose we could have tried to book an interpreter but I don't know how much easier that makes things – it would certainly add even more time'.

There are so many points for discussion from this brief scenario. I have generated a list of potential values clashes. This list, being categorised by a Western white female GP and academic with experience of working across cultures, is still bound to be ethnocentric however hard I try to consider Soraya's own values. But Box 8.1 hopefully captures some of the issues. Many of these values would be unlikely to be expressed or even admitted to if the person were asked about them – certainly we often follow the 'party line' of political correctness when discussing attitudes to people from different cultures. Note that ethnocentrism is the normal tendency of an individual to view his or herself, others and the world from the viewpoint of his or her own culture.

Exploring values and health beliefs in a culturally sensitive way

Philip mentions that he is being taught the patient-centred approach at medical school, though he hasn't heard or read much as yet about values and how important these are. So he concentrates on the patient's agenda while not realising that his values are affecting his emotions and reactions. He has suggested some of the emotions are: frustration, feeling awkward and helpless (all of which potentially mirror Soraya's feelings). He then revealed a possible disparity between this empathic approach and the media portrayal of asylum seekers as shirkers and frauds, who are out to profit from the lax British system which allows free health care to non-British tax payers.

The patient-centred and values-based practice approaches are especially relevant when there are cultural and/or ethnic differences between patient and health professional, though if a patient is from a more collectivist culture, a family centred process might be more appropriate. We also need to recognise that cultural background affects values during interactions between health professionals from differing ethnicities, religions and country of origin and training. Patient (and family) ideas, concerns and expectations are important in any consultation and should be explored by health professionals wishing to provide culturally competent health care. A major challenge might be the language barrier and, even if a person seems

Box 8.1: Conflicting values

Soraya's (possible) values

- Doctors are important people and you do what they say.
- I prefer a female health care practitioner.
- Not sure who the man is in the consultation; he looks very young – I am worried that if I say he should leave, this will affect my care.
- I would prefer to have my husband with me but he is again at some government office.
- Dealing with government officials, and even health care staff, is fraught with difficulty: I expect they will want money to help us.
- I have to behave myself otherwise I might be deported.
- I can only understand part of what is being said but I don't like to ask questions, as this nurse is obviously busy.
- Though I was given an appointment time, I assumed this meant any time in the morning – I am so used to waiting and things not happening on time.
- As I am being seen, I can also ask about my son.
- It is unlikely that these people understand anything about my religion and past life.
- It is important to have a large family and I have only one son (and one child who died as an infant).
- Some people in the UK are obviously racist and make negative comments about myself and my family.
- Sometimes I do not understand what people are saying and do not know if they are trying to help.

Philip's values

- Being patient-centred is important.
- Patients should be on time for their appointments.
- An appointment is for one person only.
- I treat male and female patients the same.
- I treat patients from all ethnicities and cultures the same, though I do not always understand them.
- I feel intimidated by women in burqas and veils – people in the UK should try to adapt to the local customs and learn the language (in time).
- These women who are covered up are oppressed and hopefully in the UK they will have more freedom.
- Some asylum seekers and refugees are trying it on.
- Some people see the UK as a soft touch due to its welfare state.
- I can't imagine what this woman might have been through.
- Why would she want another child under these circumstances?
- Is it her husband who is pressuring her into getting pregnant?
- Would she use contraception in her religion?

What other people's values might include

- These people are sponging off the welfare state.
- They are taking our jobs.
- They should be made to learn English.
- They have too many children.
- The women are downtrodden and have no rights.
- The men are sexist.
- We need to help our fellow humans regardless of their religion and customs.

proficient in English, health literacy is an additional skill to everyday conversation. However, even if language is not thought to be a problem, a patient's ideas, concerns and values may appear very different from those of one's own background and one's usual patient mix.

> **Reflection point**
>
> Health literacy is the degree to which individuals have the capacity to obtain, process and understand basic health information and services needed to make appropriate health decisions (US Department of Health and Human Services, 2000). Do you consider this when discussing health information and management with patients? Do you assume or check understanding?

In any culture there are 'old wives' tales' regarding health maintenance and medical treatments. We are aware of many of these home grown beliefs from growing up in the culture in which we then practise. However patients from other medical and health care traditions may have explanations for illness and disease that seem very strange to us and which may only be adequately explained in their own languages. These beliefs will impinge on their values. Religion also affects decisions – health professionals will be aware of the Moslem and Jewish strictures against eating pork, which may impact on what treatment is acceptable for various conditions.

Applying a patient-centred and shared decision making model may be difficult for us if the patient is from a culture where health professionals, and people in uniform, are regarded as figures of authority and thus not to be questioned. We might also have to reconsider how we approach confidentiality as family members often wish to consult together. Box 8.2 lists some of the areas that should be explored by health professionals when interacting with patients such as Soraya (noting that an interpreter may be required).

> **Box 8.2** Areas to explore in consultations (Benson & Thistlethwaite, 2009)
>
> - What the patient identifies as his/her cultural group.
> - Length of time in this country and circumstances of move.
> - Previous experiences of medical treatment in home country and host country.
> - Use of 'traditional' medicines or alternative medical practices.
> - Spiritual beliefs and how these may impact on illness.
> - Who else is involved in making decisions about health care (e.g. family, priest, religious mentor).
> - The meaning of this illness to the patient.
> - Values relating to health care practices.

Similarities between cultural sensitivity and values-based practice

Values are obviously informed by one's culture but people from the same cultural backgrounds may have different values. We notice this everyday in the UK: the variety of values displayed by UK-born citizens from similar ethnic backgrounds. Yet sometimes our stereotyping makes us assume that everyone from the Middle East or East Africa will have the same outlook on life and values. We probably recognise that there is a wide variation in how Catholics interpret their religious values, and the same is true of Moslems and other faiths. The cook book approach to intercultural relationships tends to group people by some external label and, while helpful to some extent, does not release us from exploring each patient's ideas and values. Yes, using contraception is viewed as a sin in Catholicism, but many Catholic women are on the pill; the Moslem faith abhors alcohol, but some Moslems do drink. Never assume, always ask in a sensitive non-judgemental way.

For intercultural consultations there are four possible outcomes (Box 8.3), and we can see from these that, while values are not mentioned as such, they underpin the interaction. It will be no surprise that my value is that outcome number 4 is the preferred outcome. Number 4 also recognises that the clinician has his or her own cultural influences and values and is not therefore culturally neutral. Can one ever be neutral? Philip perhaps thinks he is culturally neutral and that his values are not impacting on how he views Soraya but such neutrality is very difficult to maintain. For intercultural consultations to have a chance of being successful, the social reality of race and racism must be acknowledged (Thomas, 1995).

Box 8.3: Possible outcomes of patient–doctor interactions (adapted from Kagawa-Singer & Kassim-Lakha, 2003)

- The health professional works exclusively within the biomedical model.
- The patient and health professional function exclusively within each of their own cultures (or can substitute within their own values).
- The health professional works within the patient's cultural framework.
- The patient and health professional negotiate between their concepts of the cause of the problem/illness/disease and the most appropriate management to reach mutually desirable goals.

Overseas-trained health professionals

The scenario at the beginning of this chapter is a familiar one for many health professionals working in multicultural areas of the UK. We also need to think about the obverse situation. Recent figures show that about one third of doctors in the UK are overseas trained; there will also be other international health professionals working autonomously and in teams. Some of these practitioners will be used to consulting in a more paternalistic way than the younger generations of UK-trained clinicians. They may not be used to patients whose values include being partners in health care decisions and who might question the professional's management or judgment, or who might decline to take medicines as prescribed.

Language may also be a barrier if the clinician has difficulty understanding dialects and local idiom, leading to misunderstanding and frustration on both sides. Certainly patients in the UK expect professionals to be able to understand English and may be put off by those who struggle, which might have nothing to do with racism or prejudice.

Potential barriers to management

It is very likely that Soraya would prefer a female health professional and she may be disadvantaged if none is available. Certainly for intimate examinations, which may be required for her concern about fertility, Moslem female patients should be offered a choice of practitioner gender. Though Soraya is not fully veiled, her appearance may cause certain feelings to those who interact with her. The way patients and professionals dress may be or may be seen as an expression of their values.

> **Reflection point**
>
> Consider your own values in terms of how you dress and how you expect others to dress. This may vary depending on whether you are at work, off duty or meeting another professional, such as consulting a doctor yourself or seeing your solicitor. If someone dresses outside of these parameters how do you feel? You may dislike young women in short skirts and tight tops as much as you dislike women in burqas, but have different responses if you feel that one is making a conscious choice and the other is under peer or religious pressure. But is the young female or the Moslem woman conforming to her society's norms the most? What might a patient think about you and your public persona?

Are our cultural values underpinned sometimes by racism? 'Well of course we don't do it that way like they do over there.' And does this apply in team interactions when there are culturally diverse members?

Racial barriers in consultations and teams are difficult to acknowledge and can occur in all directions. While professionals cannot refuse to interact with people of different background, some patients may make it obvious they do not want to see a health professional of a different 'colour' to themselves. While we should not collude with such racism, if it presents a barrier to successful treatment it has to be dealt with. Cross cultural training can help the professional to raise the subject of difference in the consultation; this difference may be race, culture, gender, sexuality or even age. One suggestion on how to deal with difference is given in Box 8.4 in the words of a psychotherapist from the Intercultural Therapy Centre in London. The issue of power here is interesting. What might be the power balance in an interaction between an overseas-trained female Moslem nurse and a white British born male?

> **Box 8.4:** Dealing with difference (Thomas, 1995, page 174)
>
> 'It should be our duty to ask the clients whether or not they feel comfortable and if they are worried about the issues surrounding our race or skin colour as therapists … it is most important that therapists can give clients permission to talk about racial persecution or discrimination, since they are the people with power in the consulting room'.

Collectivism and confidentiality

Later that day Gina is asked to speak to Soraya's husband Ashraf on the phone. Ashraf's English is better than his wife's and he asks for information on what went on in the consultation. He says his wife was not quite clear about was what going to happen about the problem of her not getting pregnant and he would like to have more details. Gina answers that she cannot tell him anything about a patient without the patient's consent and that she cannot even confirm whether or not she saw Soraya that morning. Ashraf is annoyed and demands to know what is going on; he has the right to know everything about his wife's care. Gina declines to give any information and asks him to make a joint appointment with his wife to discuss any matters he has concerns about. Gina is upset by the encounter and discusses it at the next team meeting. How should the team approach confidentiality if patients have potentially different ideas about who should know what? Is medical confidentiality a cultural value?

One major professional value of Western health care practice is confidentiality. We never discuss a patient with anyone other than the immediate health care team involved in care without the patient's express permission. However such personal autonomy is not the case in many cultures. Western values are strongly rooted in notions of the individual, whereas other viewpoints are more collectivist in nature. Sociocentric communities such as those in many Eastern countries value a greater connection of the self to family, friends and the community (Draguns, 2008). Collectivism means that personal ambition is secondary to the well-being of the group (not that there is no sense of the individual in these societies). Health professionals need to be aware that, in those cultures where the self-other boundary is not so strong, patients may not see it as a breach of confidentiality if specified members of their family are privy to information (Benson & Thistlethwaite, 2009). This will usually mean husband and that there need be no formal consent from the patient. The patient's role is passive in these cases and family members are seen as the receivers of information and decision makers (Joint Commission Resources, 2006). However, like Gina, many of us will feel uncomfortable with discussing patients like this and if possible it is best to check with the patient first, explaining the values of the practice in this regard. For example, if patients require investigations you could check whether they are happy for another family member (perhaps with better English) to be given the results.

Another consequence of Western individualistic values is that many professionals, particularly counsellors and psychotherapists, use such concepts as '*self*-awareness, *self*-fulfillment and *self*-discovery' (Hays, 2008, page 47, italics added by author). Health professionals tend to expect patients to speak freely about their 'histories' but many refugees are cautious about sharing their personal information (Hays, 2008). Hays, a clinical psychologist, advises therapists she treats to consider how a particular value may affect their work with clients who may not share this value. She distinguishes between 'clinically necessary judgments' and 'judgementalism' (Hays, 2008 page 48): the former helps build a therapeutic relationship whereas the latter works against it.

The cross cultural team

Welcoming a new member to the health care team can be fraught with difficulties. We may make assumptions: as a white doctor working in Australia I am often assumed to be Australian by birth until I speak (my Northern English accent tends to point to my roots); a darker skinned doctor could have been born in Asia, metropolitan Sydney or the bush, but some patients may assume she is from overseas until they ask or she speaks. So never assume from appearance where someone might originate from – ask if necessary. It is not rude to explore each other's backgrounds if done sensitively and it might avert embarrassment and poor value judgments later on.

Refugees and asylum seekers

Soraya is a refugee and as defined by the 1951 United Nations Refugee Convention she is 'A person who is outside his or her country of nationality or habitual residence; has a well-founded fear of persecution because of his or her race, religion, nationality, membership of a particular social group or political opinion; and is unable or unwilling to avail himself or herself of the protection of that country, or to return there, for fear of persecution' (UN Refugee Agency, 1972).

While many health care teams may never have to provide care to refugees, the fact that there are approximately 20 million refugees in the world, fleeing their own country because of war, ethnic cleansing or starvation is cause for concern for us all (Kinzie, 2006). Refugees leave their country against their will and are likely to have suffered major trauma, multiple bereavements, chaos, fear, danger, torture, illness and/or starvation. They will have intimate experience of a society whose values have disintegrated or become alien to their own. While on the move, escaping from their dreadful circumstances, they will have had limited access to health care, food or clean water; have been without home, family, country, privacy or community; and been exposed to infections and injury. On making it to 'safety', they may well spend long periods of time in refugee camps, in detention or as illegal immigrants where they remain very vulnerable and often separated from other family members and friends. They will face uncertainty about the future, have concerns about deportation and may struggle to understand officials' language.

How many people under such pressure, with likely mental and physical health problems, are able to hold onto their values and maintain dignity? Over half of all refugees suffer from depression, post-traumatic stress disorder (PTSD) or anxiety disorders (Kinzie, 2006).

Refugees in a new country, which appears wealthy with good infrastructure and health care, are often hopeful on arrival but then often face rejection and prejudice that may lead them to anger, paranoia and depression (Marsella, 2007). They may suffer from culture shock in the first few months after arrival and have difficulty adjusting to the values and pressures of their new home. Culture shock is a combination of symptoms including anxiety, somatic complaints, an idealisation of the home culture (with home sickness) and even frank paranoia (Marsella, 2007). Rather than being welcomed with jobs and good housing, refugees may face suspicion. They look and sound different to the indigenous population and may be made fun of and verbally or physically attacked. Their somatic symptoms may lead to them being accused of 'putting it on' to gain sanctuary or playing the system. Many refugees have had well paid and prestigious occupations back home but these are unlikely to be recognised in their new country (Minas & Silove, 2001), making them feel once again like second class citizens, forced to take jobs for which they are over qualified. How often do we think to ask the army of foreign nationals who bolster health services as cleaners, kitchen workers or porters what has brought them to their new country, and what their expectations of their new life are? Often these hard workers are invisible to the professionals they work alongside unless they cause problems. Would you think differently of the tea lady if you knew she had been a doctor in her own country? What might this say about your values? The circumstances in the new country for these immigrants are the most powerful stressors likely to increase the risk of mental illness (Minas & Silove, 2001).

Overcoming racial prejudice by training

Health teams that interact with refugees and require intercultural skills are advised to have cross cultural and equality/diversity training, which needs to address the issues of racism and prejudice. Such training focuses on much more than acknowledging and discussing values, culture and tradition. Racial prejudice and racism are related concepts but with subtle differences in meaning. Racial prejudice arises from values, attitudes and beliefs, and is often based in misperception and ignorance, even being caused by insecurity (Fernando, 2002). Racism, however, is defined as an ideology and political stance, arising from assumptions and value judgments about inferior and superior races, combined with undertones of power and domination. Racism may arise from social conditioning and the history of a country (Fernando,

2002), its foreign policy including attitudes to invasion and colonialisation. Racial prejudice is the feeling and racism the behaviour.

Prejudice obviously is not always about race; we may be suspicious and wary of others with different values and beliefs from our own as well as being from different cultures, classes and upbringing. Possible sources of prejudice are given in Box 8.5.

Box 8.5: Sources of prejudice – adapted from Stephan & Stephan (1996) and Benson & Thistlethwaite (2009)

Source of prejudice	Effects on interactions
Negative stereotypes (cognitive beliefs)	Thinking of people from different cultural backgrounds as lazy, arrogant, prone to psychosomatic complaints, not trustworthy
Intergroup anxiety	Suspicious and hostile to outsiders and new team members, inability to understand each other
Realistic threats (economic and physical)	Belief that certain patients overuse health resources; that team members favour 'their own'
Symbolic/cultural threats	Patients and team members undermine one's own culture and beliefs

---

Race equality training aims to promote racial equality in a productive, practical and creative way, enabling participants to tackle both personal discrimination and institutional racism (Ferns & Madden, 2002). 'Race equality training must not only set up a constructive challenge to participants' personal values and attitudes but also help to develop new ideologies to support and promote equality in practice' (Ferns & Madden, 2002, page 108). 'The most important part of the training is the development of personal understanding of institutional processes that perpetuate racism, through exploration of individual feelings about issues and (more importantly) about personal professional practice' (Ferns & Madden, 2002, page 109). Institutional racism is never an advertised value of an organisation but can have a major influence on team interactions and working relationships. In the Macpherson report of the Stephen Lawrence inquiry (Stephen being a black teenager murdered in London in 1993), institutional racism was defined as 'the collective failure of an organisation to provide an appropriate and professional service to people because of their colour, culture or ethnic origin. It can be seen or detected in processes, attitudes and behaviour which amount to discrimination through unwitting prejudice, ignorance, thoughtlessness and racist stereotyping which disadvantage minority ethnic people' (Macpherson, 1999). To achieve a personal understanding of such processes means moving beyond a narrow cultural approach and the value that 'knowing about' a black person's culture, for example, inevitably leads to a non-racist stance. Participants are facilitated to consider the effects of racism on people's lives, and perhaps their own.

Working with interpreters

Philip wondered if having an interpreter would help during Soraya's consultation. Interpreters thus become part of the wider team and it is helpful to know those with whom you will be working on a regular basis. An interpreter will obviously have a very good knowledge of the patient's language but may not be of the same culture, may not have similar values and will probably not have experienced the life changes of the patient. Ideally interpreters should not only have language skills but should have relevant cultural knowledge and an appropriate professional background (Robinson, 2001) and be aware of how their values may affect their interpretation. A family member acting as interpreter is not to be recommended for many reasons including confidentiality, the need to be impartial and not affected by emotional content to the detriment of their input.

The intercultural interprofessional team

Rosedale is a sleepy country town surrounded by moors and fell land. The population is predominantly white apart from two families: one runs the Indian take-away besides the public house and one is a professional couple both solicitors in the nearby city. The general practice has three doctors, two nurses, four receptionists and a practice manager, with allied health staff based elsewhere in the town and accessed via referrals. This month the team welcomes two new members: Joshua is a GP registrar born and trained originally in Uganda, who has passed the relevant assessments to practise in the UK, and Reena is a British born Moslem and practice nurse who wears the hijab. The oldest GP, Harry Gordon, is concerned that some patients may react badly to these 'ethnic faces'. In the waiting room there is a list of personnel with photos – he wonders if patients will identity the 'difference' and what effect this might have.

> **Reflection point**
>
> What sort of orientation to the team do Joshua and Reena require? Is this different from any new member and why?

At the first team meeting after their arrival, Joshua and Reena are asked to say something about themselves, and the other members also say a few words. The youngest receptionist, Lily, is curious to know more about Reena's head scarf and why she wears it. Lily has spent most of her 21 years in the countryside and has never met a Moslem before. Her knowledge has been gained through the TV and she has images of terrorists totally at odds to what she sees in Reena as a health professional. Reena is quite happy to discuss her religion and how this affects her professional values of caring and the importance of family.

The team decides that they should discuss together how to deal with the potential situation of a patient declining to consult with a particular doctor, potentially based on appearance rather than gender. This turns out to be a fortuitous discussion as before long a patient does indeed refuse to have a consultation with Joshua. What would you have done in this situation?

Conclusion

There are moral and legal implications of working across cultures. Difficulties can arise between colleagues as well as with patients. Working with professionals from diverse cultures is helpful for our interactions with patients from similar backgrounds, however we need to be aware of stereotyping people on the basis of their race, religion or language. We know that racism is commonly expressed and encountered, usually the dominant culture having privileges compared to the weaker group. There is no place for racism within health care or within health care teams. Often courageous conversations are required to discuss values and avoid prejudice and conflict.

References

Benson J and Thistlethwaite JE. (2009). *Mental health across cultures – a practical guide for health professionals.* Oxford: Radcliffe Medical Press.

Draguns JG. (2008). Universal and cultural threads in counselling individuals. In: Pedersen PB, Draguns JG, Lonner WJ et al. (Eds). *Counselling across cultures* (6th edition). Los Angeles: Sage. p21–36.

Fernando S. (2002). *Mental health, race and culture (2nd edition).* Basingstoke: Palgrave.

Ferns P and Madden M. (2002). Training to promote race equality. In: Fernanado S (Ed). *Mental health in a multi-ethnic society.* Hove: Brunner-Routledge. p107–119.

Hays PA. (2008). *Addressing cultural complexities in practice (2nd edition).* Washington, DC: American Psychological Association.

Joint Commission Resources. (2006). *Providing culturally and linguistically competent health care.* Oakbrook Terrace, IL: Joint Commission Resources.

Kagawa-Singer M and Kassim-Lakha S. (2003). A strategy to reduce cross-cultural miscommunication and increase the likelihood of improving health outcomes. *Academic Medicine,* **78**; 577–587.

Kinzie J. (2006). (2006). Immigrants and refugees: the psychiatric perspective. *Transcultural Psychiatry.* 2006; **43**; 577–591.

Macpherson W. (1999). *The Stephen Lawrence Inquiry Report.* London: The Stationery Office.

Marsella A. (2007). Culture and psychopathology. In: Kitayama S and Cohen D (Eds). *Handbook of cultural psychology.* New York: Guilford Publications Inc. p797–818.

Minas H and Silove D. (2001). *Transcultural and refugee psychiatry. In: Bloch S and Singh B (Eds).* Foundations of clinical psychiatry. Melbourne, Australia: Melbourne University Press. p475–490.

Robinson L. (2001). Intercultural communication in a therapeutic setting. In Coker N (Ed). *Racism in medicine.* London: King's Fund. p191–210.

Stephan WG, Stephan CW. (1996). Predicting prejudice. *International Journal of Intercultural Relationships,* **20**;409–426.

Thomas L. (1995). Psychotherapy in the context of race and culture: an intercultural therapeutic approach. In: Fernando S (Ed). *Mental health in a multi-ethnic society.* Hove: Brunner-Routledge. p172–190.

The UN Refugee Agency. (1972). *The 1951 Refugee Convention: questions and answers.* Available at: www.unhcr.org/basics/BASICS/ 3c0f495f4.pdf (Accessed September 2011).

US Department of Health and Human Services. (2000). *Healthy people 2010.* Washington, DC: US Government Printing Office.

Chapter

9

A request for a home birth and other pregnancy-related consultations

This chapter considers values-based practice in the context of pregnancy and giving birth and in particular the concept of shared decision making as a component of management planning when several options are available. This is another challenging area for the team as there are often conflicts between what is considered best for the mother and what is considered best for the foetus. Moreover, the foetus is obviously not able to express any values of its own and therefore the family and health care team may act as advocates for the baby, with potential values clashes.

(Of interest is the language of obstetrics and midwifery. As a doctor I first used the word delivery as in 'home delivery' but my midwife colleague advised that birth is preferred. Deliver focuses on the action of the professional, while birth relates more to the mother. I have therefore mainly used birth in this chapter.)

Home births: a controversial option

The Moorland Surgery is in a semi-rural area of North Yorkshire. The nearest general hospital with a maternity unit is 10 miles away by a road that can be treacherous in winter ice and snow. The general practice has four full-time partners (three male and one female), two part-time (one male and one female) and currently a male GP registrar. The full-time female GP (Sheila) has an interest in GP obstetrics and, at 58 years old, has delivered many babies both at home and in the GP-led unit over 30 years. When community midwives became more autonomous, they began to carry out the majority of deliveries, though until 9 years ago it was practice policy that a GP would always be present if possible and in case of problems. The number of women opting for a home birth has substantially declined and the last one took place over a year ago. Now, none of the other doctors participate in the weekly antenatal clinic, though one is always on site doing other work and can help or give advice if needed. Sheila feels that her partners and especially the younger GPs are missing out on a key area of primary care and, though she doesn't miss the long nights waiting for babies to be born, she regrets what she thinks of as the de-skilling of doctors in some areas of practice. None of the other GPs are at all interested in intra-partum care, and indeed feel that, as they would not get enough practice, it would be dangerous for them to be involved. Sheila is aghast that delivering a baby is no longer considered a core skill to be learnt at medical school.

Julie is the community midwife who comes to Moorland most often. She has been qualified for 7 years but has never attended a home birth. She works with Sandy, who is near to retirement, a midwife who also misses the days of home deliveries.

Today Julie is consulting with Angela, a 32 year old trainee naturopath. Angela has one daughter aged 3 and is now 20 weeks into her second pregnancy. She asks Julie about the possibility of a home birth.

> **Reflection point: What are your immediate feelings?**
>
> Home births polarise opinion. Firstly try to put your emotions and values to one side and consider what you believe are the pros and cons of home deliveries. Then think how your list might be different if Sheila, Julie, Angela and one of the other doctors wrote it. Why might there be differences? Now, how do your values affect whether you are pro or con?

Personal and professional differences

Such differences will arise from what the parties concerned know about the evidence for the safety or otherwise of home births; to this they will add their own experiences of childbirth – professional, personal or both; they may have been influenced by obstetricians in the past – specialist or GPs – and their anecdotes. What is interesting here is that the values are unlikely to be split along professional lines, or even between professional and lay. There may also be those who are professionally against home deliveries but who hold the value that a woman should have a choice in her own care. Possible sets of values are shown in Box 9.1. Notice that these do not include evidence here, but some evidence could be found for many of the statements, even opposing ones.

> **Box 9.1: Possible values relating to home births**
>
> - Giving birth is a natural process, not an illness. It has been far too medicalised with too much emphasis on what might go wrong and not enough on the fact that the vast majority of deliveries are normal in this country.
> - While giving birth is a natural process, some women do want pain relief and the amount varies. Pain relief is best administered in hospital, as there is more choice and so that potential reactions can be monitored.
> - Women need to be relaxed during labour. For some women with an uncomplicated obstetric, medical and antenatal history, the most relaxing place to give birth is in her own home, surrounded by her familiar things and her family.
> - It cannot be relaxing to give birth at home because of the constant worry that something might go wrong, even if it doesn't.
> - Giving birth can be a high risk as there is always the potential for something to go wrong and therefore the safest place is in hospital, near to specialist services.
> - Midwives are the best people to assist with deliveries – they have the most experience.
> - Midwives are fine to deliver as long as there is a doctor nearby to take over if things go wrong.
> - If we had/allowed a home birth and something went wrong, we would never forgive ourselves (where we could be the family, the professionals or both).
> - Women have the right to choose, with informed consent, where they want to give birth.
> - Women should be told what is best for them and the baby and that means giving birth in hospital.
> - It is not just about the woman, there is a baby to consider.
> - I have seen too many births go wrong to consider a home delivery.
> - I have attended some wonderful births at home – they are so emotional and a great experience.
> - Next they'll be asking for water births at home and no active management of anything at all – it will all end in tears.

Home births are a difficult area on which to reach consensus by sharing values and negotiating management and by adopting an informed shared decision making process. A health professional will usually either be for or against home births, though they may say they are ok in principle (but not when I am working). It is very unlikely that an anti-home birth doctor will be swayed into agreeing with the woman's choice – so if the woman wants to go ahead with the home birth she will need to do this with a private midwife without medical back-up. On the other hand, the woman, or her partner, may be persuaded to change to a hospital birth if the evidence that is presented to them is very damning of the safety of the home option and the woman/couple are made to feel uncomfortable about their choice: you have to think of the baby; how would you feel if anything happened because of your decision? There can be a lot of guilt, and also fear, generated by such discussions.

Some professionals think that the home birth lobby is misguided and even dangerously manipulative; trying to live in a simpler era when the mortality and morbidity rate for all illness was higher and there were fewer opportunities to give birth in hospital. The home birth lobby stress that labour is natural and that the better antenatal care given to women and the ability to screen out high risk pregnancies make home births an even safer option than previously.

Health professionals may feel personal responsibility for any obstetric tragedies, and allied to this is often a fear of litigation, even if the mother has made an informed choice. So there may be an element of self-protection by the health professional, who would almost certainly be negatively affected if something did go wrong – whoever or whatever might be to blame.

Informed shared decision making (ISDM) in obstetrics

ISDM is a process that involves patient and professional reaching a mutually agreed management plan, with the professional providing evidence and ensuring that the patient has all the figures and facts with which to make an informed choice. That patients should be more involved in decisions about their care has arisen from various quarters including political trends, ethics and health service research (Kravitz & Melnikow, 2001). However, the sharing implies that the patient does not make this choice alone. There may be negotiation and compromise, so that both parties feel comfortable with the outcome (Box 9.2). Operating on the basis of ISDM rather than a paternalistic process, a health professional accepts that medical opinion is not the only arbiter of choice, that evidence and values are important, on both sides. The medical evidence may suggest a particular option is the most appropriate in terms of the general population, but an individual patient may not fall into this generality and therefore communication is important. There are a number of steps to consider in this process (Box 9.3). When no option is better than another in terms of evidence and outcomes, it is said to be a situation of equipoise (Elwyn et al., 2000) and decisions are more likely to relate to values and experience.

Box 9.2: One model of shared decision making (from Charles et al., 1997 – doctor in the original changed to health professional)

- Both the patient and the health professional are involved.
- Both parties share information.
- Both parties take steps to build a consensus about the preferred treatment.
- Health professional and patient reach an agreement on the treatment to implement.

> **Box 9.3:** The shared decision making process (Towle, 1997)
>
> - Establishing a context in which patients' views about treatment options are valued and necessary.
> - Eliciting patients' preferences so that appropriate treatment options are discussed.
> - Transferring technical information to the patient on the treatment options, risks and their probable benefits in an unbiased, clear and simple way.
> - Physician (health professional) participation includes helping the patient conceptualise the weighing process of risks versus benefits and ensuring that their preferences are based on fact and not misconception.
> - Shared decision making involves the physician (health professional) in sharing the treatment recommendation with the patient and/or affirming the patient's treatment preference.

What is the evidence?

Obstetrics is an area of health care that is very controversial and often highly political. In recent decades there have been various trends within intra-partum care driven by a number of different factors, not all of which have been solely evidence-based. To name but a few: choosing induction over starting labour naturally for convenience of either the obstetrician, the mother or both; natural child birth without medication; water births; the rising incidence of Caesarean section, including because of the 'too posh to push' trend; partners being present at the birth, and now potentially feeling guilty if they prefer to wait outside the delivery room; home births, once the norm, becoming the oddity in many countries.

There would be general agreement among the primary care team that a woman must be included in decisions about her antenatal, intrapartum and post-natal care as much as possible. In the UK a government report, published as long ago as 1993, advocated that women should have more choice in and control over childbirth. Women's choice and control therefore raised the question as to how much professional control was being lost in the process. The publication of *Changing Childbirth* (Department of Health, 1993) led to an increase in the number of home births in the UK: from 1% to 2% of all births and indeed an increasing rate of Caesarean section (Savage, 2003). However, certain decisions a woman may make are not necessarily agreed by her professional team. Moreover, even the professionals who share care (usually midwives, GPs and consultant obstetricians) may not agree with each other, causing more confusion for the woman and uncertainty as to the optimum choice for herself. For example, a woman who requests an elective Caesarean section for no appropriate medical reason is unlikely to have her choice respected in all cases, certainly within the NHS. (The cynical might say that values change if she should choose to deliver privately.) There are several reasons for this: there is an increased mortality and morbidity relating to Caesarean sections, particularly from the anaesthetic; the cost of the longer hospital stay is greater than for a vaginal delivery; recovery time is greater. However, the figures suggest that an elective Caesarean section, as compared to an emergency one, under epidural anaesthesia, with cover against the risk of thrombosis and sepsis, has not resulted in the death of a patient in the UK (Paterson-Brown, 2000). Being able to choose the date of birth, either by Caesarean section or induction, helps the woman and her partner plan when to have time off work and gives them some control over events. Updated guidelines on Caesarean section published by the UK National Institute for Health and Clinical Excellence (2011) do list as recommendation

38 that a woman who requests a Caesarean section, and after discussion still decides a vaginal birth is not acceptable, should be offered a planned section.

That differences of opinion are common in this area of practice was highlighted by a 'head to head' article in the British Medical Journal towards the end of 2011 following on from the publication of the guidelines mentioned above. Two experts were asked should a woman be able to request a Caesarean section. 'Yes' according to Turner (2011) who argued that a woman could make a fully informed decision and that women's views are important: 'their personal needs and preferences, perhaps not always fully expressed, should be respected'; 'no' according to Rouhe (2011) who argued that major surgery must be warranted. Both Turner (male) and Rouhe (female) referenced their arguments to add weight to their conclusions.

Requesting a Caesarean section may be viewed by some people in the same way as requesting a home birth. The reaction to the woman's choice can vary from flat refusal, to gentle persuasion against the procedure using selected evidence to make the points, to acquiescence with the request. The woman may have researched herself whom to consult – certain professionals will be known to favour certain approaches. Most women want to have some control over the process, and this control and decision making seems to enhance psychological well-being in the post-natal period. Most women are also sensible enough to know that things can go wrong, and that choice might need to be modified – but they want to be kept informed. There is a Monty Python sketch from the 80s: a woman in labour is being wheeled into the labour room to give birth, surrounded by doctors and machines. She asks what she should be doing? John Cleese, the head doctor, replies that she should be doing nothing – she is not an expert. We would hope that such days are gone but women still relate stories of giving birth in which they feel powerless, their labour has been taken out of their control, and there is poor communication between them and their professionals. In particular a National Childbirth Trust reporting on experiences during 2007 found that many women did not feel they were involved in decisions about their care and did not receive the explanations and information they required. In terms of collaborative care, there was often a lack of consistent advice from health professionals (NCT, 2007).

The medical narrative (the medical model) still appears to be mainly that childbirth is hazardous and therefore all labours should be approached as if they could go wrong. Yet, childbirth in the UK has never been safer (Savage, 2003). The natural childbirth narrative (social model), aligned to the home birth request, is that childbirth in developed countries is very safe and that labour should be approached as a normal event in a woman's life. These two narratives impact on values: a woman and a professional with opposing narratives are going to find it hard to reach a compromise satisfactory to both parties.

Home births were common in the UK until the 1960s: a third of women delivered at home in 1958, whereas just 1% did so in 1980 (Savage, 2003). This latter figure began to rise in the last decade and is probably about 2.5% now. Women considering homebirths may consult the British website: www.homebirth.org.uk/, which discusses the current ambiguity in the law. It used to be the case that British woman had a legal right to a *home birth service*. The local health authority was therefore obliged to provide a midwife or doctor to attend the delivery. However, while women still have this right, and a woman cannot be forced to deliver in hospital, there no longer appears to be a right to professional care. There is thus the appearance of choice, without the practical means of exercising it.

A 2009 study of home deliveries in the Netherlands covering 530 000 births found no difference in death rates of either mothers or babies (de Jonge et al., 2009). A Cochrane meta-analysis of home versus hospital birth (Olsen & Jewell, 2009) concluded that the change to planned hospital birth for low-risk pregnant women in many countries during the last century was not supported by good evidence. Planned hospital birth may even increase unnecessary interventions and complications without any benefit for low-risk women. More recently a UK study of outcomes for 64 538 women with singleton pregnancies who gave birth between 2008 and 2010 concluded that healthy women with low-risk pregnancies should be given the choice of birth setting. In particular multiparous women who planned birth at home experienced fewer medical interventions than those who planned to give birth in obstetric units (Birthplace in England Collaborative Group, 2011). Yet home birth is still very much discouraged by many midwives who buy into the medical model, whose values, and indeed training, focus on the dangers of delivery and who feel anxious about stepping outside their comfort zone of hospital-based care. When such a midwife (or indeed doctors) interacts with someone like Angela they should explain their position but also be able to discuss Angela's choice without value judgments and offer to refer her to another professional who will be able to discuss the option further.

It is interesting to consider how women form their opinions and values relating to either the medical or natural models of childbirth. For their first pregnancies, they do not have their own experience to guide them. Often anything other than a referral to hospital for care (or shared care) is not discussed. The medical model is paramount unless the woman knows there is an option. Women go into hospital to have babies. To know about other options the woman would have to have had a family member or friend discuss this with her; she may have read about choice in a magazine or online, but may not feel able to suggest this unless the health professional gives her time and space to discuss her ideas and expectations.

The midwife as a member of the team

Midwifery is a distinct branch of nursing and is a 3 year course. The professional autonomy of midwives is very variable from country to country. In the UK midwives may practise as independent private practitioners. The role and scope of practice is complex and diverse, with midwives being involved in the care of women from pre-conception, through the antenatal period and giving birth and up until about two weeks after delivery. In hospitals they work closely with obstetricians, but also practise alone. In the community they may be based in general practices and work closely with GPs and other members of the practice team, but often now they work in community clinics and communication with GPs is more problematic. Fewer GPs run their own antenatal clinics in partnership with midwives, except in more rural areas. Even fewer GPs now attend births as GP units become less common.

Antenatal screening tests

It is not only the place and type of delivery that requires ISDM but also pregnancy from pre-conception to after birth. Conception and pregnancy are natural phenomena that generate a lot of ethical debate and involve a diversity of values. Obviously contraception is not allowed under the moral code of certain religions and the termination of pregnancy is a procedure that polarises opinion from a 'woman's right to choose' to abortion's being seen as murder of the unborn child.

In the UK health professionals are allowed to exercise their consciences in relation to their own religion and not carry out operations or prescribe medication that is against their beliefs. However they are expected to refer patients onto other professionals who are willing to treat them.

Consider your own health care team. How often do we discuss our beliefs or clinical practices in relation to such issues as those listed in Box 9.4?

Box 9.4: Dilemmas around conception

- The provision of contraception to underage girls.
- Emergency contraception (and the possibility of intrauterine devices [IUDs or coils] being abortifacents when used this way).
- Social termination of pregnancy.
- Screening tests during pregnancy which may lead women to choose to abort.
- Infertility treatment provided by the state.
- Infertility treatment privately funded.
- Infertility treatment after the menopause.

Reflection point

What are your opinions on the situations in Box 9.4? Are there any inconsistencies in your thinking? What do you think would be the values of the people you work in relation to these situations?

Much of the time we are not called upon to get involved in such discussions. Do we know which of our colleagues have religious or other objections to management options that we are happy to provide? The decision about what some might think is routine care is often based on personal values rather than ethical principles, and we may be illogical in what we think is right or what we are prepared to do. For example, a nurse may be happy to prescribe the contraceptive pill to a 15 year old girl but not give condoms to a 14 year old boy.

The antenatal clinic

One of the pleasures of the antenatal clinic is that the clientele are on the whole healthy and happy women. In a rural area the women will get to know each other as their pregnancies progress and may often meet up later at nursery or childcare. Julie, the midwife, loves the way that everybody has a story; each family has a different narrative; every woman has different needs but usually similar expectations of a trouble-free pregnancy. Some are anxious about their deliveries; some are experienced and know exactly what will happen; but there are always surprises and, unfortunately, while rare there are tragedies.

Consider these four women:

Maisie Lewin is in her first pregnancy and is struggling with morning sickness. She is a 33 year old banker and used to being in control of her life. She regularly works long hours and is planning to carry on working as long as possible before the baby is born. Later, her husband will stay at home to look after their child as Maisie earns considerably more than he does. Maisie wants to have every test possible to ensure that her baby is perfect. She would also like to pick the day she gives birth to fit into her schedule, and is considering the option of an elective Caesarean section even at this very early stage of her gestation. Maisie also intends to put on the minimal weight possible and to get back to her pre-pregnancy weight as quickly as she can following the birth. She is now 10 weeks pregnant.

Lorna Chen is a 42 year old teacher in her second pregnancy. She has been married for just 1 year and conceived naturally much to her surprise. She had a termination at the age of 17 and has felt guilty about this ever since. She does not want any antenatal tests as she is prepared to have her baby regardless of any problems. She knows that there is a high likelihood that her baby may have Down's syndrome because of her age, but she and her 50 year old Catholic husband are ready to take the chance, as neither would consider an abortion.

Britney Sommers is a 17 year old, halfway through her second pregnancy. Her daughter, by a different partner, is 8 months old. Britney has always had problems remembering to take her contraceptive pill but, as she is scared of needles, had not been happy to have an implant or injection. Taking blood from her is a major effort, as she needs to lie down and not see the needle, otherwise she panics and may faint. She misses her antenatal appointments frequently and continues to smoke.

Christina Lopez is 28 and lives with her partner Anne-Marie, 45. Christina became pregnant through a sperm donor (a gay friend) and by using a syringe. Both women attend antenatal classes together and are planning a natural childbirth, preferring to have a water birth in the midwife led maternity unit, with no drugs. They have considered a home delivery but Christina prefers to be in hospital for the added safety as long as she is not pressurised to have what she would term unnecessary interventions.

Reflection point

What are your thoughts after reading the above four stories? Consider how your values and those of the women and their partners may be similar to or conflict with your own.

Four very different women; four very different stories. They, and their partners and families, will interact with many health, and possibly social care, professionals during their pregnancies. They will possibly encounter prejudice and diverse opinions about their life choices. These opinions are based on personal values intermingled with evidence-based considerations. All deserve the same level of care: but will all receive this? Even if the same team is involved in the majority of a woman's care, the team members may have very different opinions as to how the pregnancy should be managed, including place and type of delivery, use of medication, after care of the child, length of breast feeding and so on. While women are now encouraged to discuss a birth plan with a midwife early in the pregnancy, that plan should be shared with the team, as circumstances change, the plan may be altered and it becomes difficult for everyone to keep up to date. Many decisions may be made based on evidence, but that is often personal interpretation of the evidence. If a pregnant woman moves to another part of the country, will she be able to keep the same birth plan? It is rare for the health care professionals to discuss their values and their evidence base with the pregnant woman and her carers.

The four women and the team

Maisie's main midwife is also a career woman and respects Maisie's intention to work as long as possible. Her GP works part-time and has two small children. She cautions Maisie about the common difficulties associated with pregnancy that might affect her capacity to work until near term: tiredness, ankle swelling, weight gain, urinary frequency, itching; and the potential problems of any first pregnancy: raised blood pressure, premature labour etc. The midwife and the GP try to be realistic without laying on the doom and gloom, but Maisie thinks of the former as optimistic and the latter as pessimistic. While she likes the manner and efficiency of her obstetrician, who is male, she does not think he really understands working women and the need for control. However he is prepared to consider her wish for a planned delivery date but says she is likely to get over an uncomplicated vaginal delivery quicker than an operative procedure. Maisie receives pre-test counselling before her antenatal screening tests and is quite sure that she would have a termination of pregnancy if anything is wrong with the baby.

The early tests are fine but the anatomy scan at 18 weeks indicates that the baby has a missing fibula of the left leg. The radiologist explains that this is not a life-threatening condition. However Maisie says she would prefer an abortion. Her husband is not sure. The health professionals involved feel that this is an unacceptable course of action and are unsure how to deal with the request. While none of them are anti-abortion as such, they believe at this late stage in pregnancy that termination should only be considered for serious conditions likely to make life not viable or cause considerable suffering to the child. Maisie counters with – it is my right to choose and you should not force your values onto me. In this situation the team are aligned against the patient. How would this make you feel as a team member or as Maisie?

Lorna does not wish to discuss any antenatal tests. This makes her midwife feel uncomfortable as she has delivered an undiagnosed Downs baby before and remembers the devastation this caused the family. Lorna agrees to the 18 week anatomy scan as part of normal care and mainly to check that the foetus does not have any conditions that could be treated in utero. Her male GP, who is also a Catholic (a reason for her choice) is very supportive and validates her choice. He feels that undue pressure has been applied by the midwife and the hospital staff in order to make Lorna change her mind and undergo an amniocentesis. Lorna has asked if her GP could carry out her antenatal care until she is over 34 weeks as she feels more comfortable with someone who has similar values and beliefs to herself.

Often, while we do not proclaim our values, the way we speak and interact gives messages about how we do view issues. Of interest is how patients come to know of the beliefs of their health professionals, how they make choices of who to see and how these choices may vary depending on their problems. Practice leaflets do not usually define a doctor's religion, and even if they did, we cannot always infer that a health professional adheres strictly to their religious code. There may be clues in that certain doctors and nurses are listed as providing contraceptive services. Lorna knew about her GP because he attends the same church as she does but she has not asked him outright about his beliefs regarding abortion. It is his manner and support that have drawn her to him. The midwife and obstetrician have asked her at each visit about her intentions and whether she has changed her mind. This was fairly annoying, but Lorna is not the type of woman to assert herself verbally and just put up with the questions while declining the tests each time. There is a fine line between offering timely advice and pressurising people into management that they are not happy with.

Britney has everything stacked up against her: she is a young pregnant single mum who smokes. Scatty, feckless, silly, at risk – all might be applied to her. A few of the older practice staff consider her to be scheming to get a council flat – really how hard is it to use contraception properly? What sort of health professional would you be, or should be if looking after Britney. Evidence guided: she needs to stop smoking (it is the first thing you ask and then tell her at every visit), she needs more sleep; she should cut down on junk food and eat more fruit and vegetables; she is putting her baby at risk; is the father going to be involved at all? Values guided: Britney you are doing really well and I am glad you came to the clinic today. How are things? How is your daughter? Things must be a little difficult – have you got enough help? Everything seems to be going fine in terms of blood pressure and the baby's growth. Have you any concerns yourself? How is it going with the smoking? That's good that you have cut down again. Have you anything you want to ask me? Now let's think who you might want present at the birth.

Of course both professionals have values that mean they want to do the best for the baby and for Britney. Sometimes we favour some of our patients over others. We need to decide the best way to approach the health promotion problem. Being authoritarian might work for some patients, but it is unlikely to do so for Britney, who has a chaotic lifestyle and needs support. You want her to feel that she has someone to trust and to turn to if she has any questions or anxieties.

Gay couples are increasingly common, both male and female. Tact is required in consultations to ensure that the relationship of patients is clear to avoid misunderstanding and embarrassment later. Even responding to the statement 'I'm pregnant' can be fraught with difficulty for a professional. I usually ask 'Is this good news or bad' – I need to do this unless obvious from the context; even a women's verbal and non-verbal cues may be misunderstood. 'Is the father involved?' is another necessary but awkward question to avoid later difficulties. In these times of surrogate mothers, same gender partnerships, single women and IVF, the assumption that any pregnancy involves a stable male and female relationship can in itself be seen as a value judgment. Should we screen staff for sexual bias? Is anyone likely to give off the wrong signals if introduced to a same sex couple expecting a child together? What is practice policy if derogatory remarks are made?

A midwifery perspective (this section is written by a midwife colleague)

Care in pregnancy and childbirth still offers a virtually unparalleled opportunity of access to generally healthy populations seeking care. It also represents, as described in this chapter, a minefield of ethical questions, value judgments and differences of opinion. For many women and families this may be their first contact with health services and the care provided now can set the ideas, concerns and expectations that they will take forward with them. This makes it vital that in this, of all settings, individuals feel listened to, heard, involved and respected.

The four examples given in this chapter are fairly typical and, I suggest, will have resonance for many practising midwives and GPs. It is useful to have opportunities such as these to consider and reflect. What would I think? What would I say? What might I do? Why? It is this kind of reflective practice that is demanded of current professionals in health care. Yet, just as we will be steered by our own values and assumptions, we must recognise that so too will the families in our care.

How these women and their families form their opinions and values remains crucial to any discussion. Whilst one discourse remains predominant it is that voice that speaks loudest and generally gets heard. This is context specific. Whilst this chapter highlights the UK context, De Vries et al. (2007) demonstrate the 'stubborn persistence of midwifery and home birth in the Netherlands' (page 1). Without other options manifest or readily discussed it is difficult to see how women and their families will be able to absorb anything but the most common understandings of childbirth. The danger then is that most common becomes defined as 'normal'. Hence women birthing in hospital is normal, screening is normal, heterosexuality is normal and further anything other than normal is defined as abnormal. To adhere to these narrow definitions is evidently counterproductive for women, their families and care-givers themselves. Health care professionals are just as diverse as the populations they serve and perhaps increasingly so. They too are not immune to the effects of value-laden contexts and the complexities of shared decision-making.

Inevitably working in this area of medicine, as any perhaps, one's own values and assumptions will be challenged. Often this is in minor every day ways, particularly when a woman chooses to deviate from some prescribed path such as declining screening, requesting a home birth, using home monitoring equipment or requesting a Caesarean section. Whether any of this actually constitutes 'risky' behaviour or, once again, whether what is under consideration is the current definition of 'normal', is the crux of the debate. Sometimes the challenges are bigger. Care-givers have to face those 'big ethical questions about life and death' and also find a way to provide the best care possible in each, very different, situation.

So what does this mean for care providers, women and families in pregnancy and childbirth? It means that discussions and debates such as those opened in this chapter must be integral to every professional educational course and also a component that is regularly revisited in post-graduate life and every day professional practice. There is a need to make the recognition and discussion of personal values and hence the opportunities for value-based practice much more explicit. Perhaps then, balancing values in with information and evidence will become common practice. Paradoxically then it may even become 'normal'.

Conclusion

Conception and pregnancy often involve the big ethical questions about life and death, a woman's choice and the state's choice for the foetus. But there are many more minor dilemmas and decisions that are affected by the woman's values and those of the professionals in the core and wider teams.

References

Birthplace in England Collaborative Group. (2011). Perinatal and maternal outcomes by planned place of birth for healthy women with low risk pregnancies: the Birthplace in England national prospective cohort study. *BMJ*, **343**;d7400.

Charles C, Gafni A and Whelan T. (1997). Shared decision-making in the medical encounter: what does it mean? (or it takes two to tango). *Social Science and Medicine*, **44**;681–692.

de Jonge A, van der Goes BY, Ravelli ACJ, et al. (2009). Perinatal mortality and morbidity in a nationwide cohort of 529,688 low risk planned home and hospital births. *British Journal of Obstetrics and Gynaecology*, **116**;1–8.

Department of Health. (1993). *Changing childbirth*. London: Department of Health.

De Vries R, Wiegers T, Smulders B and van Teijlingen E. (2007). The Dutch Obstetrical System: Vanguard of the future in maternity care. In: Davis-Floyd R, Barclay L, Tritten J

and Daviss BA (Eds). *Birth models that work*. Berkeley: University of California Press.

Elwyn G, Edwards A, Kinnersley P and Grol R. (2000). Shared decision making and the concept of equipoise: defining the competences of involving patients in health care choices. *British Journal of General Practice*, **50**;892–899.

Kravitz RL and Melnikow J. (2001). Engaging patients in medical decision making. *BMJ*, **323**;584–585.

National Childbirth Trust. (2007). *NCT document summary. Women's experiences of maternity care in England*. London: NCT.

National Institute for Health and Clinical Excellence. (2011). CG132 Caesarian section: full guideline. Available at: http://guidance. nice.org.uk/CG132/Guidance/pdf/English (Accessed January 2012).

Olsen O and Jewell D. (2009). Home versus hospital birth. Available at: http://summaries.cochrane.org/CD000352/

home-versus-hospital-birth (Accessed December 2011).

Paterson-Brown S. (2000). Elective caesarian section – a woman's right to choose. *Progress in Obstetrics and Gynaecology*, **14**;202–215.

Rouhe H. (2011). Should women be able to request a caesarean section? No. *BMJ*, **343**:d7565.

Savage W. (2003). Professional control or women's choice in childbirth? In: Boswell G, and Poland F (Eds). *Women's minds, women's bodies*. Basingstoke: Palgrave.

Towle A. (1997). *Physician and patient communication skills: competencies for informed shared decision-making*. [Informed Shared Decision Making Project] Vancouver: University of British Columbia.

Turner M. (2011). Should women be able to request a caesarean section? Yes. *BMJ*, **343**:d7570.

10

Community-based care and the wider health care team
Professor Dawn Forman

This chapter explores how the wider collaboration of health and social care professionals works together. The number and scope of these professionals are diverse and often complex. The larger team is required for patients and their carers with multiple problems: physical, psychological and social. The greater the number and types of professionals involved, the more diverse the range of values and thus the need for collaborative goal-setting is crucial for optimum care.

While the following refers to the USA, it resonates with recent reports from the UK: 'The experiences of vulnerable older people are shaped by our basic values, including attitudes about frailty and dependence. In extolling the virtue of independence and self-reliance, the dominant culture in the United States devalues those in need of assistance, often stripping them of their power, authority and even dignity' (Olson, 2003, page 10).

Fred and Rose's story

Until recently Fred, an 87 year old, lived in a bungalow with his wife, Rose, who is also his carer. He has three sons and eight grandchildren, all of whom live some distance from the couple but whom he loves to see when they come for visits. Fred is a proud man, always smartly dressed, who has never drunk heavily and never smoked, but he does like to socialise with his friends in the local social club. Rose has always, until recently, had good health and is 7 years younger than Fred. The couple celebrated their diamond wedding anniversary last year and have photos of family and friends scattered around their home that depict the celebrations which took place at the time. Rose has however had 'a bit of trouble' with her left wrist in the last few months and has been referred to the hospital and put on the waiting list for a minor carpal tunnel operation.

For the past 20 years Fred has had a series of ill health issues and is well known to the local medical centre.

His diagnosed conditions include:

- Parkinson's disease – diagnosed when he was 67, 2 years after he retired from his engineering job.
- Prostate cancer – diagnosed 4 years ago, initially treated with radiation and now by 3 monthly hormone injections.

- Arthritis for which he had a right hip replacement 8 years ago and which also affects his knees and fingers.
- Macular degeneration of his left eye leading to poor vision and difficulty reading.

During the last 20 years, both he and his wife have been very proud that, in spite of the setbacks, Fred, with the help of Rose, has managed to live an independent life. Until 3 months ago Fred was ambulant with the help of a walking stick, was able to shower and dress and remained sociable with colleagues and friends in the local community.

Three months ago Fred suffered a stroke, which has left him with some weakness in his left side and he has aphasia, some gastric-intestinal reflux and urinary continence issues. He is able to eat an 'eat easy' diet (for example mashed potatoes, pureed vegetables and soft puddings) and again, with the help of his wife and the support of the community nurse and occupational therapist, the couple has managed to adapt at home to the new circumstances. Friends still visited and Fred continued to maintain his high standard of appearance, which included a daily shave, smart clean clothes and his favourite brown lace-up brogues.

Fred has been given various aids including a hoist, which Rose can use (if a little slowly) to help him in and out of bed and a stair lift. These have facilitated the transition back home and, with the help of a paper and pen, Rose has been able to communicate with Fred quite effectively. Both Fred and Rose have always had a high regard for the NHS and the professional people employed in the service. They feel they have had wonderful support to help them cope in their own home.

A month ago Rose was pleased to receive an invitation to attend for her wrist operation. She felt that this would help her manipulate the hoist even more effectively. She was able to communicate what would be happening with Fred and the rest of the family. Owing to the complexity of his condition, Fred was admitted into a nursing home for (as Rose and Fred understood) the duration of Rose's operation and recovery. This placement was arranged through social services.

Rose's operation went well and she returned home after only 3 days in hospital to an empty house. She realises it will take a while for her to recover fully the use of her wrist but is adhering to the physiotherapy guidance she has received and is already able to cope at home on her own. She misses Fred and has started to visit him in the nursing home on a daily basis, often staying for periods of 4 to 5 hours. She has to take two buses to get there, which takes about 1 hour on a good day. Whilst at the nursing home she carries out a lot of the duties that would normally be undertaken by the nursing and auxiliary staff, particularly helping to feed, wash and communicate with Fred.

Rose is however very concerned about the deterioration she is seeing in her husband. He is often in bed in his room when she calls and Rose is particularly shocked that he no longer seems to be taking a pride in his appearance. He does not shave unless she helps him; the clothes she finds him in when she visits often have food remains on them and his shirts are mis-buttoned. Owing to his 'minor' incontinence issues Fred has been given easy pull-on elasticised waist band trousers and wears incontinence pads. His brogues are in the cupboard and he is often wearing just his socks. Sometimes Rose does not even recognise these as Fred's socks – a few times they have not been a pair.

Rose has never seen Fred cry before, but she has recently seen tears in his eyes, and Fred certainly did weep openly when she first visited after her operation. Rose is increasingly concerned that if this continues Fred will not be fit to return home. Rose has spoken to the GP she saw recently at her medical centre; she rarely seems to see the same GP any more but the doctors are all very polite. Rose has come to realise she needs to get her points across in her 10 minute allocated consultation time, and she therefore prepares herself well for these occasions and usually feels she has made some progress after the visit, though the GPs vary in how much they will discuss about Fred due to 'confidentiality'. They do ask her about her wrist and one also enquired about her general health. Rose has spoken to various staff at the nursing home, but whilst she finds most of the staff have tried to placate her she did become quite anxious after a recent discussion with Clare (one of the nursing staff) who said, 'Well, Rose, you need to recognise that Fred is not a well man.'

After careful thought Rose therefore takes the bold step of asking her sons for help, something Fred and Rose have never done previously.

Reflection point

Fred and Rose have a fairly familiar story – the ageing couple, wishing to remain independent as long as possible. What were you thinking as you read the scenario? How do you think your thoughts are affected by your profession, and/or your experience of such a narrative in your own family? What are the likely values of the main actors in the scenario and what affects may these have on interactions and consequences? Do you know how much respite care costs for people like Fred? How do such costs affect the care that elderly patients receive?

The story from Clare – the lead nurse perspective

I am a registered adult nurse and have been working at the nursing home for 2 years. The nursing home is full at present. The management are therefore pleased. The government has decided to cut the funding to nursing homes again, and the response of the managers at the nursing home is to take on the day care arrangements from a local centre, which is closing. This increases the work load and whilst more day staff have come to the nursing home they are not 'up to speed with the way things are done around here'. I am the lead nurse for Fred and 15 other clients but of course I work shifts and am not always here on site.

Fred has complex needs. I really appreciate Rose's coming as regularly as she does as Rose helps out a lot during the time of her visits. However I do feel at times that Rose is being unrealistic about what Fred can do and cannot do. I have no doubt in my mind that Fred has done very well to remain independent for so long and feel he really should have been in the nursing home before this. Now he is here, I don't think that Fred will be going home again. I have great difficulty however in getting Rose to realise this and I am not keen to push the conversation too much in this direction as I want Rose to keep visiting and helping Fred in the way she has been doing. I have a slight concern that Rose may 'make a fuss' when she does realise Fred will not be going home.

To protect myself and to ensure that I have been seen to be keeping a record, I have written down my observations of Fred's full condition, his lack of mobility, his inability to communicate, his incontinence, his medication and of course factors around what I have diagnosed as his 'depression'.

The story from the perspective of the nursing home GP – Dr Turner

The nursing home has become increasingly busy during my weekly visits. It is impossible to make a full assessment of each person's progress. GPs take on the care of nursing homes in their community and practice area and, while some of the residents may already have been registered with my practice, there are many I do not know as they have lived outside this area before moving here. In the case of Fred he is not a regular patient of mine as his home is several miles away across town.

Each patient is, of course, seen once a week, though this may be a brief encounter if the nursing staff report no change in the resident's condition. A more thorough assessment of each patient is undertaken on a monthly basis. These tasks usually fall to me unless I am on leave. Sometimes our GP registrar visits on my behalf. At the practice we have a new GP registrar twice a year. Some are really interested in elderly medicine and some find it hard going to interact with nursing home patients with multiple conditions. Every 6 months a report is made of the patient's progress by the nursing staff, and every year the nursing home GP tries to meet with the family together with the patient and nursing staff to discuss and develop an on-going management plan.

It is very difficult for people to get into a nursing home as community and primary care facilities try to support patients in their own homes for as long as possible but, once in the facility, there is very little likelihood of their going back to their own home again. Many families are relieved when their relatives move into a nursing home and often visits from relatives are at best spasmodic. Usually it is children who place their surviving aged parent into a home. Some of these children seem to want to do this as cheaply as possible. Some want the best care but do not visit, and some are very caring and supportive: this indicates very different values about family responsibility and duty.

Fred is relatively new to the nursing home and has only had one full assessment. Fred has complex needs and there is no doubt he has done very well to remain in his own home environment for so long. Clare indicates that unusually Fred's wife is visiting on a daily basis and helps out quite a bit with Fred when she is there. Understandably, however, Fred has difficulty communicating and this, together with his other conditions, means he is confined to his room most of the time. The symptoms of Fred's Parkinson's disease, his stroke, etc. are under control. At Clare's suggestion I also added medication for his depression to the cocktail of pills he has already been prescribed. I am always reluctant to prescribe sleeping pills for elderly patients because of the risk of confusion and falls. Fred is often drowsy during the day and Clare says he can be awake most of the night according to the night staff. Hopefully the antidepressants will help improve his sleep pattern in the next few weeks. Fred's mobility is limited and, whilst a visit from the physiotherapist or occupational therapist may be helpful, with Fred's communication difficulties this seems unlikely. Clearly with Rose visiting so often it might be useful to both Rose and Fred to obtain a speech therapist's opinion and management to aid communication and to see if any improvement can be made with Fred's eating and drinking. Clare has asked if I could talk to Rose but Rose is not around at the time of this assessment, so maybe next time.

The perspective of the youngest son – George

Mum really seems upset. I have phoned the nursing home and made a bit of a fuss so they have called 'an exceptional case conference' next week during half term. I will be up for the week and will see both Mum and Dad prior to the case conference and see what can be done.

The perspective of Julie – the speech therapist

What a lovely couple Fred and Rose are. Rose is really keen to help her husband and Fred seems to light up when Rose walks in the room. After all those years together it is wonderful to see. Rose is doing a great job with the pen and paper and I have added the 'point to pictures' mechanism to support what she and the nursing staff are doing. It is doubtful however that the nursing and auxiliary staff will have much time for this. Nevertheless Fred and Rose seem to like the idea. Adjustments can be made to Fred's diet. He loves Rose's trifle and enjoys Jaffa cakes. Fred seems to be able to manage these and at 87 why not give him a treat? For the nursing home meals and drinks minor modification is recommended, along with a small amount of thickening agent for Fred's drinks. Whilst the nursing home does not have them, Rose has managed to get hold of a fork/spoon combination I recommended, which seems to be really helping Fred to eat more independently.

It is unusual for the speech therapist to be called to the case conference but it will be a good experience. I am looking forward to it.

> **Reflection point**
>
> What are your thoughts having read the scenario? What do the actors' statements say about their values? Do the values and behaviours match?

The theoretical perspective applied: values and behaviours

The case of Fred and Rose is not unusual. There are approximately six million carers in the UK, of whom nearly a half are over the age of 50 (Carers UK, 2011). These carers often feel guilty when they have to give up caring because of their own health, change in circumstances or deterioration in their dependant's condition.

Whilst each individual professional has acted appropriately in the case of Rose and Fred, all the staff are busy. In this new nursing home environment not only do the professionals not know Fred and Rose and their history but there is little time to understand them as people and little time for communication between all of the staff involved in overseeing Fred's care. There is no continuity between the care Fred and Rose have had in their home environment and that of the nursing home and, whilst Rose has almost a 'blind faith' that health professionals will do what is best for both of them, she is not aware of the other political pressures the individuals may be under. She is increasingly concerned about Fred's condition and when he will be coming home. In the scenario no personality difficulties between the individuals or difficulties in understanding professional boundaries have been identified but each person seems to have different patterns of behaviour and perhaps different values.

When explaining from a psychological perspective the way a person behaves, and the relationship of their behaviour to their values, it is often helpful to think of the layers of an onion (Figure 10.1).

The behaviours a person exhibits are a function of their relational skills; their ability to communicate easily and to both see and manage conflicting views; their knowledge and professional or personal skills and abilities; their underlying attitudes and beliefs; and their fundamental ethics, values and convictions.

As indicated earlier in this book, the importance of shared values being clear and understood if an organisation is to function effectively and have sustainability was first recognised in private sector business (Peters & Waterman, 1982; Austin & Peters, 1985). Since this time many organisations include the values and beliefs of the organisation in their strategic and corporate plans and aim to ensure all employees and service providers know of, agree and demonstrate these values in their day to day activities.

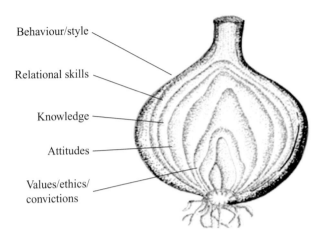

Figure 10.1. Model of relationship between values and behaviour (adapted from De Haan and Burger, 2004). Reproduced with permission of the author, Centre for Coaching, Ashridge.

Behaviour/style

Relational skills

Knowledge

Attitudes

Values/ethics/ convictions

If we try to summarise what may be the underlying values, attitudes and beliefs relating to the people involved in this story, perhaps the following may be appropriate:

Fred

- A proud man.
- With Rose's support, independent.
- Likes social interaction but ones which he can control.
- Holds the NHS professional staff in high regard.
- Wants to be at home.

Rose

- Loving.
- Caring.
- Supportive.
- Always puts herself second.
- Family oriented.
- Holds the NHS professional staff in high regard.
- Quite astute in her dealings with her own GP and the professional health care staff she encounters.
- Wants Fred to be home where the family can care for him as they should.

Clare

- Efficient; above all else Clare wants to be seen as efficient.
- Would rather adhere to than challenge a bureaucratic situation.
- Fearful of the possible consequences of her actions and how others in the team will judge her.
- Conscious of the cost cuts in both the nursing home service and the NHS.
- A little sceptical about the care that can be achieved in the home.

- Caring but feels the professionals, including herself, know best.
- Does not like confrontation.

Dr Turner

- Busy, does not have the time to check up on past records and really get to know the individuals in his care and is frustrated by this.
- Conscious of the politics of the NHS and the nursing home.
- Recognises he has the ultimate responsibility for the patient in his care and therefore is concerned about not having the time to ensure the rest of the people in the team undertake their roles appropriately.
- Keen to be seen to be doing a good job but conscious of the costs of bringing in changes and additional opinions.
- Has always enjoyed interacting with the elderly.
- Feels a little uncomfortable about all the medication and the subsequent polypharmacy consequences, which are needed by patients in the nursing home.

George

- A proactive person who wants to be seen as caring and moving things forward.
- Supportive of his parents but torn between what may be best for his father and what may be best for his mother.
- And also considers what is best for his own immediate family (wife and children).

Julie

- Seems interested in the person as a whole although her professional ability is limited to speech therapy and swallowing.
- Really cares and indeed admires Rose and Fred.
- Wants to do what she can to improve Fred's condition.
- May be prepared to bend the rules if it means making a difference.

The dysfunctional team

As noted in Chapter 2 there are many definitions of 'team', with the recurring theme of members linked through having a common purpose. Teams are especially appropriate for conducting tasks that are high in complexity and have many interdependent subtasks.

In this scenario the common purpose is the care of Fred and to a lesser extent Rose. Each individual, including Fred and Rose, has an interest in the care that Fred is receiving. Currently, however, they are not working together with common understanding and common goals. They are therefore not working as a team. The team, which does have a common purpose, could be said to be dysfunctional in our case study. In an acute hospital environment, health care professionals are encouraged to share information about a patient. Increasingly these hospital environments are encouraging the 'team' working with the patient to be interprofessional and to take on board the views of the patient and carer or relatives. There is however some progress to be made in this regard.

The individuals (including Fred) are not working as a team. The 'team' of people with an interest in Fred's care is therefore dysfunctional. As we saw in Chapter 2 (page 76, Box 2.5)

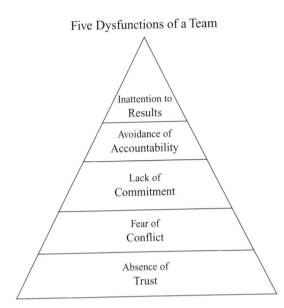

Five Dysfunctions of a Team

Figure 10.2. The dysfunctional team (Lencioni, 2002, p. 188). Reproduced with permission from the Table Group, Lafayette, California, USA.

Lencioni (2002) outlines five dysfunctions of a team (Figure 10.2). We can review each layer in turn as to how it applies in the case of Fred.

Reflection point

Before reading on consider how the team is dysfunctional. Do you think that the health professionals involved in the scenario consider themselves to be a team? Do you agree that Fred and Rose are part of the team? Do you feel that the health professionals involved consider Fred as 'the patient at the centre of the team'? If you were asked to work with this team to help it function more effectively, what would you do and why?

Absence of trust

We have considered trust a number of times particularly in chapter 7.

'Essentially, this stems from their unwillingness to be vulnerable within the group. Team members who are not genuinely open with one another about their mistakes and weaknesses make it impossible to build a foundation for trust' (Lencioni, 2002, p. 188)

With the team involved in Fred's case there is almost a blind trust from Fred and Rose as they

- Hold the NHS professional staff in high regard.

Others in the team however are more sceptical for example:
Dr Turner

- Recognises he has the ultimate responsibility for the patient in his care and therefore is concerned about not having the time to ensure people in the rest of the team undertake their roles appropriately.

Clare

- Fearful of the possible consequences of her actions and how others in the team will judge her.

Perhaps more understanding of each other's roles and values would help to build the trust which is needed for the team to work effectively.

Fear of conflict

'*Teams which lack trust and fear conflict are incapable of engaging in unfiltered and passionate debate of ideas. Instead they resort to veiled discussions and guarded comments*' (Lencioni, 2002, p. 188).

Clare in particular seems to want to avoid a conflict situation and is doing her best to ensure she is adhering to the expectations of the management team of the nursing home rather than to the needs of Fred or Rose. It is in Rose's nature not to make a fuss and to believe the professional staff will do what is right, but with support from her son she is at the point where she wants to tackle the situation even if this may cause some conflict. However, many patients and carers may feel powerless in a conflict situation and are also concerned that 'complaining' may make matters worse. To deal with this fear, the first step is to acknowledge that conflict may well be productive. Avoiding conflict to lessen the risk of hurting others' feelings, because one values harmony for example, may only allow dangerous tensions to build up, that eventually need to be resolved in a potentially more harmful way (Lencioni, 2002).

Lack of commitment

'*A lack of healthy conflict can lead to a lack of commitment. Without having aired their opinions in the course of passionate and open debate, team members rarely, if ever, buy in and commit to decisions, though they may feign agreement during meetings*' (Lencioni, 2002, p. 188–9).

Dr Turner has little time to review Fred's situation and no real time to meet with Rose. Clare does not want conflict and avoids raising what she sees as the only logical prognosis for Fred. As yet there has been no first meeting but hopefully, if appropriately organised, real agreements can be reached and not just 'feigned' agreements.

Avoidance of accountability

'*Without committing to a clear plan of action even the most focussed and driven people often hesitate to call their peers on actions and behaviours that seem counterproductive to the good of the team.*' (Lencioni, 2002, p. 189).

In Fred's case there has been no clear plan of action agreed by the team. Indeed no real plan at all and each individual has their own view of the goals to which they are aiming.

Inattention to results

'*Occurs when team members put their individual needs (ego, career development) or even the needs of their divisions above the collective goals of the team*' (Lencioni, 2002, p. 189).

In the case of Fred there has been no attempt so far to clarify what everyone hopes to be achieved by his care. The team has not yet met as a collective, and the views of the 'patient'

Fred and his carer Rose have not been heard or understood. Little or no attempt has been made to understand Fred as a person and what he really values and wants for his future.

> **Reflection point**
>
> Lencioni (2005) advocates a step by step approach to overcoming the dysfunctions of a team. How can the team in our case study, which has the common purpose of Fred's care, learn to:
>
> - Trust one another?
> - Engage in unfiltered conflict around ideas?
> - Commit to decisions and plans of action?
> - Hold one another accountable for delivering those plans?
> - Focus on the achievement of collective results?

How this case study could be used

There are a variety of ways in which this case study can be used to stimulate discussion of the patient and client needs in a care environment (and see Chapter 15 for more discussion of learning and teaching of values-based teamwork).

As a starting point the case could merely be used to open discussion with regard to:

- Whether a 'team' should exist in this scenario and if so how can the dysfunctionality of the team be remedied.
- Whether working with a shared set of values would be appropriate.
- At the very least, how the individuals involved could share expectations and communicate more effectively.

Role play

The case study could form the basis for role play where professionals actually gain experience of what it feels like to be Clare, Fred, Rose, George, etc. and thereby enhance their understanding of the impact of care and the different contributions and concerns the individuals have.

Facilitated interprofessional discussion

The case study could be used with students on interprofessional programmes, workshops for professionals, in house training etc to ensure the care of the client as a whole is considered.

Resources

The above learning situations can be enhanced using one or more of the following techniques:

- Kleine, N. (1999). *Time to think*. The technique outlined by Kleine ensures each individual has both the opportunity to express their views and time to think and be listened to in an appropriate way.
- Thomas, K. W. and Kilmann, R. H. (1974). *Conflict Mode Instrument*. This technique invites the participants to consider how they communicate and how they deal with conflict situations where different perspectives can be quite challenging.
- Myers Briggs MBTI Handbook (Briggs, M. I. McCaulley, M. H., Quenk, N. and Hammer, A. (1998) or techniques such as Vilkinas, T. and Cartan, G. (2006) *Integrating*

Competing Values Framework which provides each individual with the opportunity to gain greater understanding of their own values and priorities and how those may differ from those of their colleagues'.

References

Austin NK and Peters TJ. (1985). *A passion for excellence: the leadership difference.* London: Collins.

Briggs MI, McCaulley MH, Quenk N and Hammer, A. (1998). *MBTI handbook: a guide to the development and use of the Myers-Briggs type indicator (3rd edition).* Mountain View, CA: Consulting Psychologists Press.

Carers UK. (2011). Available at: www.carersuk.org/newsroom/stats-and-facts (Accessed December 2011).

De Haan E and Burger Y. (2004). *Coaching with colleagues: an action guide for one-to-one learning.* Hampshire: Palgrave Macmillan.

Kleine N. (1999). *Time to think: listening to ignite the human mind.* London: Octopus Publishing Group.

Lencioni P. (2002). *The five dysfunctions of a team: a leadership fable.* San Francisco: Jossey Bass.

Lencioni P. (2005) *Overcoming the five dysfunctions of a team: a field guide for leaders managers and facilitators.* San Francisco: Jossey Bass.

Olson LK. (2003). *The not-so-golden years: caregiving, the frail elderly and the long-term care establishment.* Lanhan, MD: Rowman and Littlefield.

Peters TJ and Waterman RH. (1982). *In search of excellence: lessons from America's best run companies.* New York: Harper Row.

Thomas KW and Kilmann RH. (1974). *Thomas Kilmann Conflict Mode Instrument.* Tuxedo, New York: Xicom.

Chapter

11

Ageing and end of life decisions

This chapter explores the interplay of values and teamwork in end of life care.

There are many big ethical dilemmas about end of life and palliative care. As the population of many countries ages, euthanasia is a topic that is constantly in the media, while conditions in the UK's aged care and nursing facilities are undergoing much scrutiny. Elderly patients and clients are frequently cared for by teams of professionals, whose individual members may have different values relating to prolonging life or hastening death. The team caring for a dying patient is hoping to provide a 'good death' and members may become emotional and vulnerable. Any existing team dysfunction may be magnified at such emotive times.

As we age, we begin to consider what our future holds. We value the right to die with dignity while realising that, while we may be fortunate and die in the place of our choosing, we are unlikely to be able to choose the time or manner. Health professionals share this ultimate experience with all their patients as we are all aware we are going to die, and therefore we may expect that we can empathise with the emotions that such knowledge brings. There may be denial, fear, acceptance, readiness, happiness, sadness, anger, powerlessness. As with other areas we have explored, professionals have personal and professional values, that may be conflicting, that may conflict with others in their team, that may conflict with the patient's and their family's. More people are considering whether it is their right to choose a time, manner and place of death. Some British citizens exercise that choice by travelling to Switzerland to die with *Dignitas*, while in the Netherlands euthanasia is sanctioned by the state, under strict conditions. While we may rarely have to grapple with major ethical issues, day-to-day discussions about life and death are influenced by values amongst the team and held by patients.

Reflection point

What are your values in relation to end of life care? How do you stand on euthanasia? Do you understand the terms active and passive euthanasia? Do you know if any of your team members are pro-euthanasia? How many of your team consider it is a health professional's responsibility to try to heal and comfort and not to hasten death under any circumstances? Is it important to have these conversations with your team? How might you approach discussing the topic?

Inquiring about advance decisions

A few months ago John and Margaret Fitzsimmons consulted Dr Brian Ellis, their GP of 20 years, about the possibility of making an advance decision (see Box 11.1). At the time John, 73, and Margaret, 76, were in good health. John was on no regular medication and Margaret was taking one tablet a day for mild hypertension (ramipril). The couple wanted to discuss their options about end of life care and medical interventions while fit and mentally competent. Neither relished the thought of becoming a burden on the other, or on their two daughters. John explained that he was in fact an advocate of voluntary euthanasia while Margaret disagreed with active hastening of death but did not want treatment to prolong her life if its quality were poor. Dr Ellis had some experience in this area and was able to point his patients in the direction of appropriate legal advice and eventually the required documents were signed with copies being placed in the medical records. John and Margaret had some concerns that circumstances in the future might mean that not all health professionals involved in their care would either know about their wishes or feel able due to personal or professional values to uphold their decision. In particular they raised the question of how any hospital-based health professionals would know about their advance decisions if they were admitted to secondary care when ill. Dr Ellis therefore decided to discuss the topic of end of life care and patient autonomy at a practice meeting. He realised that he did not know how many of the practice's patients had advance decisions nor what some of his colleagues thought about them.

Box 11.1 Advance decisions

In the UK an advance directive (also known as a living will but unlike standard wills does not involve money or property) is now more commonly known as an advance decision.

People can make an advance decision to refuse medical treatment in the future if they became unable to make their own decisions, i.e. have a lack of capacity. The directive should include the particular treatment they do not want such as CPR (cardiopulmonary resuscitation), blood transfusion, intravenous fluids. This refusal relates to all treatment not just that which is thought to be life-saving. It is a legally binding document in England and Wales. The advance decision cannot be used to request specific treatments, assisted suicide (which is illegal in the UK) nor refuse treatment for mental health problems.

While not mandatory, it is advisable that advance decisions are drawn up by a solicitor to ensure that they are valid. Instructions should be specific to avoid ambiguity.

For further information see: www.direct.gov.uk/en/Governmentcitizensandrights/Death/Preparation/DG_10029429 (accessed December 2011).

Dr Ellis's experiences over the years had shown him that there is a huge variation in people's attitudes to death and dying, what they think they might want at the end of life when they are well and what they actually want when they are terminally ill. Health professionals too have different values. Added to this complex mix is what is legally and ethically allowed in a country and how customs and practice change over time. Moreover an agreement between patients and professionals in primary care may not be known, or may be ignored, if patients are admitted to hospital. Sometimes family members do not always know what their loved ones have decided, or do not agree with the decision and conflict may arise.

Reflection point

What do you know about advance directives and their legality? Should a health professional ever be pro-active about discussing a patient's end of life plans? And if so at what age should this happen? Perhaps you have discussed dying and funeral arrangements with your parents. What did this feel like? Is it your responsibility as a health professional to ensure that your elderly patients have had these discussions with their family?

Values relating to the end of life

This is a time when values are still often influenced by religion and morality. But in an increasingly secular society, many factors also come into play. A person's race, religion and culture may not completely signpost how they will react to their own impending death, or that of someone close to them. As with many other areas of practice, health professionals bring their personal values to their work, tempered by their professional values and legal obligations. Some may not disclose their personal values if they are outside what is considered the mainstream of care, which for many culminates in preserving life at all costs.

Patients are particularly vulnerable when severely ill and unable to make informed choices for themselves. They rely on professionals and carers, but also on having their previously expressed wishes about the level of medical intervention respected. The last thing that is necessary is the team, including carers, having conflicts over management. In some cases legal advice is also sought by one or more parties, adding to the complexity of the decision-making process and potentially deferring decisions about outcomes.

The discussion about advance decisions at the meeting was fairly sedate. Some of those present did not know much about them; most of the GPs had had some patients inquire about having one. The practice manager said that some time ago it had been agreed to enter the existence of advance decisions in a patient's notes as a special code in the computerised records. Hardly anyone at the meeting remembered this. The team decided not only to revisit using the code but to have a register of patients with advance decisions that could be referred to as necessary. They also agreed that when referring patients to hospital, mention should be made about the decision and what it contained, and that the patient, or more appropriately the carer as the patient would be incapacitated for the decision to be used, should be informed that this had been done.

A more difficult discussion about euthanasia

While everyone was feeling satisfied with the agreement reached about advance decisions, Paula Tomlinson, a recently qualified GP, recalled an experience she had had while a GP registrar in another practice. A terminally ill patient, Annie, had asked advice about going to Switzerland for euthanasia. The patient, with breast cancer and spinal secondaries, was in a great deal of pain. She had been given a prognosis of between 3 months and 6 months left to live but did not feel that she wanted her condition to decline further. Annie wanted control over the time and manner of her death and her partner, Lily, was prepared to assist in getting her across Europe. Paula had been very upset by the conversations with the two women. As a junior doctor she had strong values relating to helping patients and considering her patients' ideas and concerns, but had not thought of helping them to die. Her values, affected by her ethics training and her learning of the four basic moral principles (Beauchamp & Childress, 2001), highlighted the importance of beneficence and non-maleficence. (The other two principles are autonomy and justice.) In some respects she felt that doing no harm was stressed more than doing good.

Paula's GP trainer, a practising Catholic, advised her to treat the case like abortion – not to hinder the couple in their decision, but not to support it actively with encouragement. Moreover, unlike abortion, Paula did not need to refer her patient to a professional who would agree with euthanasia, as euthanasia is not legal in the UK. Paula also spoke to a palliative care nurse working in her practice area, who recommended that Annie visit one of the local hospices to see that many patients were able to be cared for through a 'natural' death without pain. Paula could find no-one within her practice, or in the young GPs group of which she was a member, who would advocate for the Swiss *Dignitas* solution, or at least admit that this was a possible course of action. Paula asked: 'Surely if we value being patient-centred, and work to involve patients in decisions about care, we should be able to discuss options with them that we might find distasteful but that are still options open to them. I should not be enforcing my values on the patient by abdicating any responsibility'. Brian Ellis raised the question of what we mean by a 'natural' death in these circumstances and does our use of the word natural in certain circumstances relate to our values?

At the meeting there were 10 health professionals and the practice manager. Their spread of opinion and questions raised are shown in Box 11.2 and definitions relating to the topic are in Box 11.3. All agreed that even with the best facilitator in the world, the team would never reach consensus on the issue, and perhaps this should not be expected. So how best to tackle the decision as to what might become practice policy? Should there be a practice policy or should it be every professional for him or herself? Should patients be informed of what the different team members think? In other words should we try to ensure that patients' and professionals' values agree before certain consultations?

Box 11.2: The spread of opinion on euthanasia

- Preserve life at all costs – do nothing to hasten death and use medical science as much as possible to keep someone alive.
- It is the health professional's duty to preserve life but we do not need to use heroic measures to prolong it artificially *(raising the question as to what is meant by heroic measures)*.
- We should neither encourage nor discourage patients from choosing euthanasia abroad – it is their decision.
- We need to debate euthanasia more in this country but for the moment it is illegal and therefore I will not be involved in any discussion about it.
- I think euthanasia should be legalised similar to the Dutch model, with appropriate safeguards.
- Terminally ill patients should have choice over the timing of their deaths but I could not hasten a patient's death: someone else would have to do it.
- Whose values are more important for end of life decisions? The patient's or the professional's?
- I would not like to think that health professionals were discussing how and when I should die even if I can no longer make the decision myself.
- We are able to decide when beloved pets are put to sleep out of love, why not our human loved ones?
- Murder is illegal and ethically wrong. Why are we even talking about this?
- What if a carer wants euthanasia for their relative, but the relative is not able to agree?
- I hope that by the time I am in this position, I will be able to be assisted in dying if I request it.

Box 11.3: Definitions relating to euthanasia

- Euthanasia is the active killing of a patient by a physician, on the patient's request and in the patient's interest (Dupuis, 2003, p. S61).
- Voluntary euthanasia refers to killing a patient at their request while non-voluntary euthanasia is the decision to kill a patient who lacks capacity to understand and therefore cannot give meaningful informed consent (Kerridge et al., 2005).
- Active euthanasia involves giving a patient a treatment that directly and intentionally kills them while passive euthanasia is the withdrawal or withholding of a life-saving or sustaining treatment (Kerridge et al., 2005).
- Physician-assisted suicide is when the doctor provides the means or gives information that enables a patient to end his or her own life (Foley, 1995).

Interestingly, the GP registrar Jan van Basten, had trained in the Netherlands, where a law permitting both assisted suicide and euthanasia came into effect in 2002 (Box 11.4). However, euthanasia had been discussed and practised in the country for at least 25 years before. Jan reported that an act as controversial as euthanasia becoming legal does not alter people's values systems. Those doctors who had previously agreed with the process now had the right to carry it out, while those who did not would not become involved. The Netherlands law focuses on what might be called a doctor's professional value to ease suffering. According to Dupuis (2003) the strongest and most undeniable argument in favour of the law is the principle of tolerance, and that autonomy of the patient overrides non-maleficence on the part of the doctor. Besides it is the patient who is deciding that in his or her case no harm is being done. 'Why shall we burden each other with our personal views on life, illness and dying? Why is it not possible to accept that people have different opinions about the real personal issues of life and death? Why not accept a moral plurality concerning the end of life? This is the real issue that every society with highly advanced medical care has to reflect upon. Tolerance is of course not the ultimate value, but it could be so, when actions of individuals have no or limited consequences for others' (Dupuis, 2003, pS64).

Box 11.4: Aspects of the law from The Netherlands (see www.healthlaw.nl/wtlovhz_eng.pdf – last accessed December 2011)

- The law in the Netherlands requires that the doctor terminates a life or carries out an assisted suicide with due care and that this is done in a medically appropriate way, thus the acts become medical treatments.
- Euthanasia is allowed for patients with a lack of capacity for making their own decisions.
- People qualify for euthanasia or assisted suicide if the doctor believes that the patient's suffering is lasting and unbearable – the condition does not need to be physical and the patient does not need to be terminally ill.

Hastening death – a dilemma

The meeting moved on to consider values relating to hastening death rather than euthanasia. The participants felt that this was not as clear cut black and white illegal because such an action can be considered as within acceptable medical practice. However each patient's story is different and so are the reactions of health professionals in diverse circumstances. End of life care is likely to be the responsibility of several professionals working together due to its complexity. There is therefore the potential for conflict and misunderstanding of actions. The law relating to treatment, non-treatment and futility (the concept relating to the burden of treatment being out of proportion to any possible benefit) is convoluted and health professionals are advised to seek legal advice from their indemnity or professional bodies, or local ethics committee, if in doubt.

The case of Arnold was discussed as an example of how differences between colleagues may manifest. Arnold Pettifer is an 87 year old man with worsening heart failure who lives alone. His wife died of bowel cancer 11 years ago. Arnold has always been an active man. He was cycling on the country roads up until 8 months ago when he started to develop shortness of breath. Even then he continued to walk to the village newsagents for his daily paper until 2 months ago when he had a mild heart attack. He had declined to be admitted to hospital and is being looked after at home by a team of health professionals including the district nurse, who visits twice a day, his GP who visits weekly and as necessary, a night nurse he pays for himself who sleeps over at his house every night and a nursing attendant who bathes him three times a week. He has meals on wheels and his only daughter, Polly, a 59 year old laboratory worker, stays with him most weekends.

Arnold says his main problem is boredom. He cannot leave the house unless in a wheelchair when his daughter comes and takes him out, but many weekends the weather is too bad. He doesn't much like the TV and finds his eyes hurt after a few hours; reading is also difficult for longer than an hour or so due to macular degeneration in his left eye. He has the radio on for large parts of the day, alternating between music and talk. His legs are swollen and he has a painful ulcer on his right foot due to a fall. He has told his daughter he is just waiting to die. His daughter has broached the subject with GP Dr Rajanake as to whether her father might be depressed. Might he benefit from antidepressants? The doctor, however, feels that Arnold's mood is perfectly understandable given the circumstances and that Polly is feeling helpless with the need to have something done. He presumes she feels guilty not being able to stay with her father the whole time.

Nurse Susan Fletcher wishes she could spend more time in the house but she has a heavy workload. Arnold often tries to engage her in longer conversations but she tells him she has to get on. Arnold has also told Susan that he wishes someone would put him out of his misery. The nurses check that he is taking his medication but he often asks what is the point. He has had a good life and is ready to leave the world. Susan has also told Dr Rajanake that Arnold uses the word misery to describe his condition, but that when they do have a chat about the world, Arnold is quite animated and engaged.

This scenario is becoming more and more common as patients live longer, and are therefore more likely to go into a slow decline, having to give up pleasures and diversions, their lives becoming restricted to their homes. At the meeting at least one of the health care team would be prepared to help Arnold die, but this person does not admit this to the group. We do not always feel able to share our values if we consider they would not be understood or endorsed by other team members or professionals. We may speak in general statements (I can certainly see situations where it may be preferable to help someone to die if they wished it) but not in particular cases (I consider that Arnold has the right to die if he chooses and I would help him).

Reflection point

What are your thoughts about Arnold's case? How would you feel if Arnold were your patient? A family member? Yourself? Even consider how you would feel if your 15 year old dog or cat had become housebound, needed to be carried outside to go to the toilet but still appeared to enjoy being stroked. What differences do these circumstances make and why?

More about Arnold

Is Arnold depressed? The answer to this depends on how we view depression in this instance: as a state of mind, a medical illness or the rational response to a deteriorating situation. Arnold knows he is not going to get better. The pleasures of his life have all been taken away apart from his daughter's visits, but she is miserable herself because of his condition and yet is continually telling him to 'cheer up dad'. So he is unhappy at his lot and he is ready to die. So in one way we could say that his depression would be cured by his death.

Who else would gain from his death? His daughter would financially but she does not need his money as such. She hates the thought of being an orphan, of having no blood relatives in the world. She is divorced and has no children. Her father alive and ill is better than her father dead. Is she being selfish? However she has no way of helping him die.

By the way: Polly herself is under a great deal of strain. Occasionally when she meets one of the health care team at her father's house, they ask how she is doing. But the main focus is Arnold. Polly loves her father but on occasion she does consider that her life would be better if he were in a home or even if he were to pass away (she would not admit this to anyone).

Each reader of this scenario will have slightly different values in relation to what could and what should be done about such patients. Some of our values might conflict: I want to help Arnold but the way to help him is against the value I place on life. The team rarely meets as a team – they communicate via the patient records left at the house, or by the phone. The doctor is requested to visit by phone and he sometimes calls when one of the nurses is at the house. People behave with efficiency. They get the job done. They talk to Arnold and make sure he has what he needs but they try to avoid hearing the request that Arnold has. While Susan has mentioned Arnold's mood to Dr Rajanake, they have not had a conversation about his death wish nor have they discussed this with Polly.

> **Reflection point**
>
> Would you recommend a team meeting about Arnold? If so, now consider who should be present at such a meeting: would you include Polly and Arnold himself? Perhaps you feel a trial or antidepressants may be helpful. What may be the advantages and disadvantages of such a course of action (if Arnold consents to take more pills)?

The final episode

While Dr Rajanake is Arnold's most regular doctor, sometimes one of the other local GPs is on duty when a visit request comes in. Dr Smith calls one evening a few weeks after the practice meeting when end of life issues were considered. Arnold has complained of chest pain. Dr Smith last saw Arnold about three weeks ago and feels that he has aged considerably in that time. He has lost weight and his muscles are wasted. Arnold's pain tonight appears to be muscular rather than cardiac but Arnold asks for something for the pain. 'It is really severe doctor.' Dr Smith has morphine injections in his bag – he wouldn't hesitate to use this if he thought Arnold was having a heart attack and then would admit him to hospital. He also has some strong codeine tablets (30 mg). He is unsure what to do. The night nurse arrives and he therefore asks her to give Arnold two of the codeine tablets to help his pain. He leaves another four tablets besides Arnold's bed and advises him to take another two if the pain wakens him during the night. Arnold dies later that night in his sleep; the nurse is unable to wake him at his normal time and notices that there are no codeine tablets left. The nurse puts in a complaint to the surgery that Dr Smith's actions caused Arnold's death. She feels that Arnold should have been admitted to hospital rather than left with inappropriate analgesia for undiagnosed chest pain.

Reflection point

What are you feeling about this now? What are the characters' reactions likely to be and what should happen next?

Of course Arnold might have died anyway that night. How did the codeine contribute? Some might say that Arnold is better off – he has what he wanted and is now at peace. Did Dr Smith act with the right motive, i.e. wanting to ease Arnold's pain? Is motive enough or is the outcome of the action what needs to be judged? Could Dr Smith have given morphine and justified his actions by saying that the chest pain could have been ischaemic and therefore an injection was the right treatment? Polly has had only admiration for her father's care up to this point. Is she likely to want to take action in her grief?

The team will possibly be divided over the next move. As the senior doctor Dr Rajanake calls a practice meeting to discuss what happened as a significant event audit (see Chapter 4). However, the night nurse is from an agency and is not part of the local primary care team. Should she be invited? She has now made a complaint to the primary care organisation and is waiting for an investigation. Who will benefit from such an investigation? Dr Smith's notes from his visit will be very important. Meanwhile Susan feels guilty that she considers that Arnold is now better off. He died in relative peace in his own bed.

This story has no clear cut resolution. I imagine a team of dedicated health professionals circling around Arnold's home, nipping in and out with relatively little interaction. Arnold was at the centre of these circles and was perhaps lucky by some standards in having his own home, a caring relative and the ability to pay for extra support. There are differences in how communities value its elderly citizens and decide on the resources required to support them.

Caring for the elderly

Peter McLintock, age 85, and his wife Joan, age 76, live in a small house in the town of Waverley. Peter has vascular dementia and Joan no longer feels able to look after him. He gets up frequently during the night and wanders about the house, waking Joan who worries that he will fall and hurt himself. When she tries to get him back into bed, he is often abusive to her and thinks she is a stranger. The couple has been married for over 50 years and Joan feels guilty about considering putting Peter into a home for the elderly mentally ill. Their oldest two children and five grandchildren are supportive of this move and have been liaising with social services and the mental health community team to find a suitable place for Peter. Their youngest child, Barbara, is a teacher and divorced and has offered to move into the family home to look after both her parents. This would entail her giving up work and relying on a carer's allowance, the couple's pensions and savings as income. She would also rent out her own flat. This suggestion receives a mixed reception. Joan does not want to be a burden on her family, but she also does not want Peter to be 'locked away' in a care facility, especially given the recent stories in the media about cruelty and neglect. Joan talks over her dilemma to practice nurse Kay when she has her annual influenza injection. She also discusses the problem with her GP, Dr Malik, a practising Moslem whom she has known for 15 years.

Reflection point

What are your thoughts about care of the elderly? Do your personal and professional values clash? Have you ever suspected or had to deal with elder abuse? Perhaps you have had to consider future plans for ageing relatives of your own or dealt with patients/clients with aged dependents. Can you think of possible cultural differences and how these may relate to cultural values in the above scenario?

In an ideal world our parents would live to a ripe old age in good physical and mental health, die before their children in their own home without suffering, having lived a good life and died a good death. Unfortunately, not many elderly people do have this good fortune. Many are left alone by the death of their partner, have no children to care for them and require help with the activities of daily living. How a society treats its aged citizens reflects its underlying values; but what it espouses are not always what takes place. Care of the elderly is an expensive business and how much of that expense the state will pay varies between countries and governments.

In the UK we have the strange situation that in Scotland health and social care for the elderly is free at the point of delivery, whereas in England social care is means tested, and the definition of where social care ends and health care starts depends on location. In many countries without any form of welfare state, families are expected to look after their elderly relatives and indeed consider it their duty to do so. What is clear is that the proportion of the population over the age of 65 is increasing and that during the next 10 years the number of people over the age of 85 will double (Dunnell, 2007).

In the scenario of Peter and Joan, if we consider the possible values of the family members and the professionals, we will probably find dissonance between the values expressed and the behaviour displayed (Box 11.5).

Box 11.5: Values relating to elderly care

- Children have a responsibility to look after their aged parents just as their parents looked after them during childhood.
- Ageing parents may need specialised care best given in a care home or aged care facility.
- The state should pay for aged care if the elderly person has paid taxes all his/her life.
- Elderly people should pay for their own care until their finances run out at which point the state should pay.
- Children should expect to inherit their parent's wealth rather than it being used to provide care.
- It is morally wrong to put aged parents in a home if they have a child to look after them.
- Children should not be expected to look after aged parents as they have to consider their own lives and the needs of their own children.
- We do not value the wisdom of our elderly citizens enough – we should treat them as valuable assets in our society.
- The elderly are neglected and not looked after properly in care homes as staff do not care and are not trained properly.
- I would rather die than end up in a care home.

We may expect that Dr Malik, being a Moslem, is from a culture with the tradition of the extended family, perhaps three generations living together to provide support, child and then elderly care. This is of course a generalisation but in a multicultural society as health professionals we will interact with clients who consider care homes for the elderly as an abdication of responsibility.

A colleague's comment (a health visitor, end of life researcher and interprofessional educator)

There is no avoiding dying – it is perhaps the only certainty in life – but knowing when, where and how we will die will remain a mystery. So perhaps it is only right that we debate the issues that this brings – the personal views we each hold of what we would want and what we may believe or view as a 'good death', how we view life and living, will all serve to influence that which we believe to be right. Whilst each one of us will hold a different perspective of this, influenced no doubt by our personal beliefs and values, our upbringing, our experiences – what we will perhaps be united in is our wish to die without pain and with dignity.

Working within our chosen health and social care profession places an obligation to listen to each person's voice – to hear what is being said and to try to understand their perspective. Evidence suggests that most people want to die at home with their loved ones near and without being a burden. Dying in this way is only possible if the health and social care professionals work together and with the dying person and their relatives. Everyone has one chance to get it right – get it wrong and relatives can be left with memories tinged with guilt, horror and anger. Get it right and relatives are left with memories of sadness and loss but also peace and acceptance.

Dying at home requires the input from district nurses, social workers, occupational therapists, general practitioners, specialists (nurses and doctors), health and social care assistants, voluntary and statutory agencies. Each has a separate, but important role; each professional's decision has an impact on another team member. Effective and frequent communication is essential and key to understanding and supporting. Exploration of other perspectives is essential if we are to be able to provide support and reassurance at times like these.

Conclusion

The area of end of life and aged care is a values-laden part of professional practice. Health professionals need to be aware of the legal and ethical underpinnings of what they do, may do and may not do. Their work and interactions will be affected by their values and those of their patients and colleagues. Our society may change in how it views end of life decisions in the future, driven by the values of the majority of the population, but these decisions may well conflict with those of the minority.

References

Beauchamp TL and Childress J. (2001). *Principles of biomedical ethics*. New York: Oxford University Press.

Dunnell K. (2007). The changing demographic of the UK national statistician's annual article on population. *Office for National Statistics*. Available at: www.statistics.gov.uk/articles/population_trends/changing_demographic_pictue.pdf (Accessed December 2011).

Dupuis HM. (2003). Euthanasia in the Netherlands: 25 years of experience. *Legal Medicine*, 5;S60–S64.

Foley K. (1995). Pain, physician-assisted suicide and euthanasia. *Pain Forum*, 4;163–178.

Kerridge I, Lowe M and McPhee J. (2005). *Ethics and the law for the health professions (2nd edition)*. Annandale: The Federation Press.

Chapter

12

Referrals and the interface between primary and secondary care: looking after 'our' patients

This chapter explores the referral process of patients and clients between one health professional and another, in particular considering the referral from primary to secondary care but also between professionals in the community. We consider the concept of continuity of care and responsibility, plus teamwork in hospital.

In those countries such as the UK and Australia where traditionally general practitioners have a gatekeeper role, the majority of patients' first interactions for health problems and health maintenance take place in the community. The European definition of a general practitioner from 2002 is a doctor who provides both comprehensive and continuing care to every person seeking medical care. This definition stresses that first point of medical contact within general practice and the nature of the care provided in that GPs deal with all health problems (Wonca Europe, 2002). However over the last 10 years the nature of that first contact has changed. Thus the first health professional consulted could be the individual's GP, but it could also be a pharmacist, a practice nurse or nurse practitioner, an allied health professional or a complementary therapist. However, to access secondary care or hospital-based specialist services, patients still require a referral from a GP. The one exception to this is if patients access Accident and Emergency (the Emergency Department) directly.

A patient moving between primary and secondary care faces certain challenges. The secondary care team provides treatment when the patient is in hospital. Sometimes the boundaries of this team are difficult to define: there may be multiple small teams and a loose collaboration of other health professionals depending on the nature of the patient's problem (Box 12.1). On discharge, a full record of what happened during the in-patient stay should be communicated to the patient's general practice as soon as possible including arrangements for follow-up and any community-based care that is required. A patient, who is seen or followed up in out-patients, is still also under the care of the GP and it is easy for care to become fragmented. Patients may receive conflicting advice when undergoing investigations and/or treatment from multiple sources. The notion of teamwork, and even collaborative care, becomes very fluid in such circumstances.

Mrs Meldrum is admitted to hospital

Felicity Meldrum, a 74 year old woman, is admitted to hospital by her GP because of an exacerbation of her chronic obstructive pulmonary disease (COPD). Felicity did not want to be admitted as she knows that people often pick up nasty infections on hospital wards, but she lives alone and is too breathless at present to be able to look after herself or get to

---

Box 12.1: The hospital team

Medical team	**Nursing team**	**Other health professionals**
Consultant/specialist	Senior nurse	Pharmacist
Registrar	Staff nurse	Physiotherapist
Foundation doctors	Nursing students	Occupational therapist
(Medical students)		

Wider medical team	**Wider team**	
Radiologist	Radiographer	
Pathologist	Laboratory assistant	
Microbiologist	Ward clerk	
	Medical secretary	
	Social worker	

---

the toilet alone. Her GP Dr Simon Birch would have liked to have put in place a 'hospital at home' type care arrangement, but there is a lack of trained community-based staff able to do this at the moment due to sickness and recent resignations. He promises Felicity that she should be home in a few days.

Dr Birch, like many GPs, prefers to look after his patients at home if possible. His primary care values are such that he believes that patients should have the choice of care at home or in hospital unless their condition is such that only hospital care is appropriate. He knows that many elderly patients, like Felicity, are concerned about the standard of care in hospitals, including the potential to acquire nosocomial infections and the lack of attention from hard pressed nursing and medical staff. Dr Birch is a partner in a practice that shares these values: it is difficult to practise in this way unless the doctors, and primary care team, agree that patients should have the option. Looking after sicker patients means more frequent home visits, being on call for the practice's patients out of hours and being able to rely on the whole team for the necessary skills and responsibilities.

Dr Birch admits Felicity to hospital with some apprehension, but also does believe that she will be cared for appropriately. While she is in hospital he feels that he is giving up his responsibility for her. If there was a community or 'cottage' hospital he would have been able to continue to provide care but such hospitals are rare in the UK now. GPs do not tend to visit their patients in hospital; he could ring up to see how she is doing but most likely he will only know what has happened to Felicity when he receives a discharge note from the admitting medical team, or if he is informed that she has died.

Primary and secondary care collaboration

Primary care and secondary care teams are only loosely affiliated to each other. Communication tends to be at the beginning and end of episodes of in-patient care. If a GP has been working in an area for some time, he/she will know the hospital specialists and have formed an opinion of their capabilities, both interpersonal and technical. Similarly the specialists get to know the 'good' GPs in their patch. However for an admission, Dr Birch might speak to a junior doctor who is taking admissions, or even a bed manager depending on the local situation. Such conversations can be difficult – the junior doctor might be trying to preserve the last medical admission bed, the GP does not like his or her clinical judgment about the necessity for an admission to be questioned. All the health care professionals would probably say they have similar goals and are patient-centred but they do not always interpret patient-centredness in the same way. For an admission the GP is focused on his or her patient; the admitting officer is focused on the work load, bed situation and the patients already in the hospital.

Mrs Meldrum in hospital – the worst case scenario

Felicity is on the medical ward and is being treated with intravenous antibiotics for what has turned out to be community-acquired pneumonia. She is poorly but expected to recover. Dr Birch has included in his referral letter that she is allergic to penicillin and this has been recorded in her notes. Unfortunately 5 days after admission she has a mild stroke affecting her left side and has difficulty swallowing. She has a brain scan and is started on the appropriate treatment. For a while no-one is monitoring her calorie intake – she can use a fork and spoon with difficulty but cannot manage some of the food that is put in front of her. The ward orderly who is responsible for giving out meals removes them again uneaten, without the nursing staff being aware of what is happening. Felicity then develops a urinary tract infection (UTI), which results in her being very confused. She is moved to another ward with a higher staff to patient ratio. The new team looking after her are not aware of her pre-morbid personality, that she lived alone in her own house without help before admission. They see a confused elderly lady and treat her, with all good intentions, like a child. Moreover the UTI is treated with amoxicillin (a penicillin) due to an oversight and Felicity comes out in a very itchy rash. Her worst fears are realised.

Eventually after 8 weeks Felicity is discharged home, having lost a lot of weight, her confidence and her mobility. The discharge note gives a medically orientated story of the admission which does not prepare Dr Birch for the lady he sees when he visits her at home the day after she returns. Before admission she was on two inhalers and now she is on several drugs, most of which she does not know the names of or what they are for. A daily home visit from a community nurse has been arranged. Felicity is able to get about the house, but with some difficulty and she has lost her vitality. She is happy to see Dr Birch, whom she regards as 'her' doctor. Dr Birch is saddened by this episode, but knows that without a full story of the course of events, it is hard to blame anyone. The hospital has a statement of its values on its website but these cannot always be upheld if there is a shortage of staff, staff retention is poor, morale is low and handover is sub-optimal. He wonders if he should speak to anyone in the hospital hierarchy to express his concerns, but doubts it is worth the effort. He feels that he can only ensure that his own team in primary care functions well.

Reflection point

Felicity's story is the worst case scenario; unfortunately we do read in the papers frequently about the lack of care in some hospitals and the adverse events arising from this. Do you consider that Felicity's problems are related to poor team work? What other factors have precipitated her deterioration? Which could have been prevented and how?

Continuity of care: my patients or the patients?

In the above scenarios I refer to Dr Birch in relation to Mrs Meldrum as 'her' GP. Dr Birch probably has referred to Mrs Meldrum as 'my' patient. Both pronouns refer to possession. In this case Mrs Meldrum may have one GP but Dr Birch has over one thousand patients on 'his' list. Strictly speaking in the UK now, where a high proportion of GPs' remuneration is from capitation fees, i.e. an annual amount for each patient registered, patients register with a practice rather than a specific doctor. Some patients are happy to consult with any doctor in 'their' practice; some like to consult with only the one they identify as theirs: my doctor. This relationship is an interesting one. In previous decades, and when UK GPs had a 24-hour responsibility for their registered patients, the notion of 'my patients' was very real. Though the responsibility might be shared amongst a practice's several principals, there was a sense of the GPs working together to cover out-of-hours and handing back the patient the next morning. Single handed GPs did not have that choice and could truly refer to my list, my patients. Many GPs delivered a baby, looked after her with measles, prescribed contraception when the baby was a teenager, looked after her ante-natally and delivered her baby in turn. Continuity of care meant that a GP knew a family, not only the medical history but also the social and psychological as well. Such continuity was a value of British general practice and was defined as care from one doctor usually spanning an extended time and for more than one episode of illness (Freeman, 1985). Now I would suggest that we say that it is care from one team, with an assumption that the membership of the team is fairly stable. There are a number of types of continuity now recognised (Box 12.2). One of the most difficult aspects, as I have stressed throughout this book, is the owning and sharing of the information. Information that encapsulates a person's whole life story is rarely written down and, if it is, it is rarely completely available at these moments of cross over from one professional to another. So, the patient is asked to recount their story over and over again.

Box 12.2: Types of continuity of care (adapted from Freeman & Hjortdahl, 1997; Haggerty et al., 2003)

- **Longitudinal care:** given by the same health professional over a defined time (can refer for example to a GP or hospital specialist).
- **Personal continuity:** an ongoing therapeutic relationship between a patient and health professional; the health professional (usually a doctor) is viewed by the patient as the most valued source of care; quality of contacts more important that quantity.
- **Informational continuity:** the use of information on past history and personal circumstances to make the current care appropriate for the patient; requires accurate, complete and up-to-date medical records.
- **Management continuity:** a consistent and coherent approach to the management of a patient's health condition; responsive to the patient's changing needs and wishes.
- **Relational continuity:** an ongoing therapeutic relationship between a patient and one or more health professionals.

Reflection point

What values do you hold in relation to continuity of care? How accessible should an individual health professional be to 'his' or 'her' patients?

Even before the 24 hour responsibility was passed over to the local primary care organisation to arrange medical cover out of hours, and long before walk-in centres enabled people to see a GP or other health professional without being registered, many practices began to join co-operatives or pay private firms to provide out-of-hours cover. The co-operatives were groups of GPs from a local area who covered for each other's patients, meaning that the chances of a patient having their own doctor visit at night were greatly reduced. Handover of patients following a night visit was no longer face-to-face but via phone or even fax. GPs moved from the value of continuity to the value of work-life balance. And I am not making a value judgment here: doctors who are up at night dealing with sick people and emergencies do not function as well the next day, when they were usually expected to work. So a doctor could be out of her bed three or four times a night to deal with anything from a child with a temperature to an elderly person in heart failure. Then back in surgery at 8.30 am the next morning having had at most 3 hours sleep. From personal experience I know this makes one irritable, less empathic and more prone to take short cuts and hence make mistakes.

Even so when a doctor admits a patient to hospital, it is usually with a sense that he is sending in his patient: My patient (or my partner's perhaps) is being given over to the care of another team of doctors and health professionals. I trust them to do the right thing. Sometimes they don't.

Patients also refer to 'my GP': 'I need to make an appointment with my doctor', though increasingly this may be substituted by: 'I need to go to the doctor's' or 'I need to see the nurse'. During the multiple crossings of the interface between community and secondary care patients may also state that they have an appointment at the hospital or with the specialist, sometimes they may indeed refer to 'my specialist'. A patient's navigation through the care system is now often referred to as a patient's journey. This journey usually relates to a single condition such as cancer but patients are more likely to have several conditions as they age which overlap in time. This is particularly the case for people with chronic disease or long-term chronic conditions such as diabetes, heart disease and arthritis. Individual patients have different ways of dealing with this. Some regard their hospital physician as the 'person in charge'; others look to their general practitioner as the repository of knowledge about their condition. Increasingly there may also be a nurse specialist who spends most time with the patient and family.

Reflection point

What is your experience of how are decisions are made within an extended health care team or collaborative? What makes the process work well and what hinders effective collaboration?

A referral to secondary care

Doctors refer patients to other health professionals regularly. When referring to a specialist within the secondary care setting, a GP does this for one of several reasons (Box 12.3). In this sense the care is now shared between the two doctors. If a different medical problem arises while the patient is being seen at out-patients, the general practice will deal with it. While an admission might almost be seen as loaning a patient to the hospital for care, out-patient referrals are not a temporary abdication of responsibility.

While there might be a specific reason for referral, GPs do not always make this clear. Thus patients referred for initial management of a chronic disease may stay in the hospital system for a while, seeing a specialist once every 6 months or so, when in fact their GP is perfectly capable of carrying on treatment and monitoring. It is important in the referral letter to state what exactly is the nature of the help being requested.

A referral from a doctor to an allied health professional also has its own etiquette. In the majority of cases these referrals follow diagnosis and specialised treatment is being requested.

> **Box 12.3:** Reasons to refer to secondary care
>
> - Unsure of diagnosis – requires investigation/specialist opinion.
> - Diagnosis known – requires special medication not available in primary care.
> - Diagnosis known – requires specific management (e.g. ante-natal/delivery, radiotherapy).
> - Diagnosis known – requires surgery.
> - Patient asking for second opinion.
> - Family requesting second opinion.

However the allied health professional, such as a physiotherapist or speech therapist, has a much better knowledge of the treatment options available, so a referral should include the diagnosis (tentative or firm) but not a specific course of therapy, allowing the allied health professional leeway in this regard. It is possible that a physiotherapist or other professional may disagree with the doctor's diagnosis: the two health professionals should then discuss this and come to a consensus. Both then learn from each other's knowledge and skills. There is no place in the system for a doctor to dismiss another health professional's opinion without a respectful discussion: we can all be wrong at sometime.

Valuing and respecting each other as professionals

Mark Quinlan, a 42 year old policeman and experienced marathon runner, consults his GP James Kenny one evening. He complains of a pain in his right calf for the last few days, which is worse on walking, but pain free when resting and at night. Mark is in training for the London marathon and has been increasing his weekly mileage over the last few weeks. He had run 20 miles the day before the pain started. James examines Mark's calves and finds no swelling, redness or local tenderness. The pain is worse when James extends and flexes his right ankle. Mark says he thinks it is just a muscle sprain but wants to exclude a stress fracture or other more serious condition. James reassures him, saying that he also thinks this is a sprain. Mark says he will make an appointment to see the physiotherapist he can access via work as he does not want to stop training for too long.

Two days later James is left a message to ring sports physiotherapist Colin Lynott about their mutual client Mark. Colin had rung earlier and asked to speak to him but James was in the middle of a consultation. The receptionists know that James does not like to be interrupted when seeing patients unless there is an emergency. James tries to get hold of Colin at the end of his busy surgery but Colin is then treating one of his clients. Eventually after several tries by both men, James speaks to Colin after 5.30 pm. Colin has seen Mark, who said that not only had he pain in the calf but that his foot was intermittently feeling cold. Colin had examined Mark's feet and legs and could find no peripheral pulse on the right side. He wonders if Mark has an arterial blockage of some kind.

> **Reflection point**
>
> What are your feelings at this point of the story? How might James, Colin and Mark be feeling? What would you now do if you were James?

James is feeling a mixture of guilt, irritability and embarrassment. He is irritated not by the fact that Colin has rung him to suggest, in the most respectful way, that the GP's diagnosis is incorrect, but that he has to make a decision about what to do at this hour of the day. He should see Mark, not only to examine him and possibly refer him to hospital, but also to re-build his confidence, which may be dented if Colin has suggested there has been an error. James is also irritated because he realises he could have dealt with this much sooner if he had taken the first phone call, but it is a value of his not to short change his patients by taking calls during consultations – he does not like to try to multi-task. Colin has been in situations where doctors have been quite rude to him if he suggests an alternative diagnosis to theirs. His responsibility is to the patient and he is prepared to take the time to contact the doctor and to bear the brunt of any rudeness in order to give the best care. He has also been careful not to suggest to Mark that James may have made a mistake – he has suggested that something may have developed that he would like checking. It will be up to James to discuss any potential error with Mark.

When James examines Mark he agrees with Colin's diagnosis and makes sure that Mark sees a vascular surgeon urgently. He rings Colin later in the week to thank him for his clinical acumen and to let him know what is happening. Colin is pleasantly surprised by this; while he feels that James should have picked up the problem, he admires the fact that he is able to speak to Colin about the outcome and recognises that they are both working together for the good of their patient/client.

Reflection point

Have you any experience of one professional either praising or insulting another in relation to the management of a patient's case? Perhaps this has happened to you. What does this say about values? Even if someone makes a mistake in relation to 'your' patient, is this the correct way to behave? What should you do?

The case of Sarah

Sarah Bolt, a 46 year old mother of two, has not been feeling herself for a few months. She initially presented to 'her' GP (the doctor who she has seen most regularly at the practice for contraception and post-natal depression) with vague symptoms of bloating and lower abdominal pain. She had not lost any weight, felt tired and anxious. Her older daughter (just 16) had been diagnosed as 24 weeks pregnant the previous month. Dr Rose examined Sarah, could find no abnormal signs in her abdomen and queried whether it was the stress of the daughter's concealed pregnancy that was affecting Sarah. The symptoms worsened during the pregnancy but Sarah did not see Dr Rose herself again until her grandson was a few weeks old. By this time she felt she had lost weight. Dr Rose now wondered if Sarah could have ovarian cancer and referred her immediately for an urgent ultrasound scan and specialist opinion.

The scan was highly suggestive of cancer. After the registrar had listened to Sarah's story at the gynaecology clinic he said it was a pity her doctor hadn't referred her earlier. The symptoms she described were highly suggestive of ovarian cancer. Sarah was shocked and in her delicate psychological state, began to blame Dr Rose for her predicament. Though the registrar did not say it in so many words, she assumed that the late diagnosis would adversely affect her prognosis. She decided she did not want to consult Dr Rose again and began to see another GP in the practice.

Reflection point

What do you feel about this narrative? There are a number of possible responses (Box 12.4). What does your response have to say about your values?

Box 12.4: Responses to the story of Sarah

- Dr Rose and the registrar are theoretically on the same team – they need to respect each other.
- The registrar should have considered that making a negative criticism of a colleague is not warranted and that this will not help Sarah's relationship with her GP.
- The registrar does not know all the facts: ovarian cancer is notoriously difficult to diagnose.
- Sarah has been let down by Dr Rose and she is right to feel angry.
- Sarah has been let down by an offhand remark of the registrar and she is right to feel angry.
- Sarah should make a complaint against Dr Rose.
- Sarah should make a complaint against the registrar (or at least tell his boss).
- The registrar was quite right to say what he did.

We often make disparaging remarks about our colleagues, or perhaps indicate to patients by our body language that, in our opinion, their care has not been optimal. While we may think this, we need to be sure we have all the facts before acting in a negative way. Of course, if it really is the case that care has been substandard, we should take action. But think back to the case of Felicity, what should we actually do?

The primary–secondary care interface

Health professionals interacting with patients need to explore with patients (and their carers as appropriate) who is also currently providing advice and treatment. When a patient is admitted to hospital, the admitting doctor, nurse or clerk (as appropriate) should always ascertain who is the patient's GP or practice. However, just as frequently no-one asks the patient about their over the counter medication or complementary therapies, it is likely that there will be no specific inquiry about the patient's other community-based health care professionals and complementary practitioners other than their registered practice. It is also possible that it may not be known that the patient is already under the care of hospital specialists, if he or she is now being admitted to another hospital. The potential for fragmentation, duplication and confusion is high. This, of course, could be alleviated with patient held records, or universal records, accessible from anywhere within the national health system. Patients may remember names and places, but when ill and under stress, may forget specific details.

Health professionals, when exploring what patients understand about their condition (ideas and concerns), should find out where the patients have gained such information from: their GP, the Internet, or perhaps their midwife, community psychiatric nurse, chiropractor or friend. These clinicians and lay people use different language and concepts to describe illness and disease mechanisms. Moreover the patient filters and makes sense of this language, based on his or her experience or values. If a professional dismisses any of this knowledge from the patient's trusted sources, even denigrates it either verbally or through body language, the patient–professional relationship will get off to a bad start, and the patient may not listen to the professional's information and advice. Or they may begin to question the previous advice and lose trust in their sources, causing problems when discharged.

At the interface there is a delicate balance between trust in the old and setting up trust in the new relationships. A throwaway line, such as in the case of Sarah, may do lasting harm. Moreover, sometimes a professional's subconscious values affect communication, though he/she may not always be aware of this. If a professional thinks that chiropractic is 'quackery' and a waste of money, or that homeopathy lacks evidence, then she is unlikely to consider that any positive therapeutic effect that the patient describes is important. Patients may recognise this scepticism and become reluctant to talk about their complementary therapies in the future. There needs to be a dialogue about the treatment so that patients do not dismiss the opinions of their orthodox care providers and not adhere to management plans which conflict with what they already believe.

Reflection point

Should health professionals respect patients' choices even if they feel they are unhelpful and lack an evidence-base? What would you do if your patient asked your opinion about crystal therapy, acupuncture, homeopathy, HPV vaccination, meditation, becoming a vegetarian? How may your advice and opinion be affected by your values? And your understanding of your patient's values?

Our professional responsibilities

It is a health professional's duty to take action, which may involve informing the relevant accreditation body, if they have concerns about a colleague's performance or fitness to practise. The General Medical Council (GMC) states in *Good Medical Practice* that doctors must protect patients from risk of harm posed by another colleague's conduct, performance or health (GMC, 2006). Within a workplace there need to be reporting procedures in place. Obviously such referral is only taken after due consideration and discussion within the team and with the person concerned as appropriate.

Reflection point

Have you ever considered referring a colleague for poor performance? Do you know the procedure for this, particularly if the colleague is from another profession? Your intrinsic values may rebel against 'telling tales' or 'dobbing someone in'. How do you cope with this conflict?

Teamwork in hospital

Hospitals are full of teams – what grouping of professionals classifies as a team depends on how they work and function together (as discussed in Chapter 2). Many departments and specialties have regular and effective multi-disciplinary team (MDT) meetings, to discuss patient care and team performance. How teams work in such large and complex organisations is the subject of research in social science, business and health care.

Colleagues of mine in Australia have recently completed a research grant enabled series of reports for hospitals looking at communication in emergency departments (ED). They used ethnographic and other qualitative research methods to explore the interactions of the ED staff (Manidis et al., 2009). There is not room here to go into great detail but I will highlight some of the main findings in the context of values-based practice.

At one of the hospitals, between eight and fifteen staff were involved in a patient's care. One patient, whose face-to-face interactions with staff lasted 47 minutes in total, had 62 separate encounters in that time. While a number of different professionals were involved in care delivery (mainly doctors and nurses of various grades), there was very little interaction between them at the bedside and few interprofessional handovers. This resulted in the information gathered about and given to the patient becoming fragmented. One of the recommendations arising from the report was the development of effective inter-disciplinary team work and organisation of care.

Clinicians, who incorporated patient-centred approaches in their practice, such as using inclusive language, being empathic, expressing personal attitudes and *values*, and interspersing interpersonal chat with medical talk, were rated more positively by patients. Health professionals identified a tension between their professional clinical practice (and therefore values) and the professional management culture (and its values). Clinical practice focuses on the relationship between patient and professional, while management focuses on system requirements such as waiting times and patient flow.

Similar results have been found on hospital wards in Singapore. Again this research used observation and interviews with health professionals to look at communication but this time on medical, surgical and intensive care units. Nurses interacted with nurses much more than with doctors, and vice versa: only between 0.7% and 7.6% of interactions were between doctors and nurses. This project used social networking methods to capture the interactions. Nurses and doctors communicated with patients on separate occasions rather than together, again raising the possibility of fragmentation of care and duplication (Lim, 2011).

A patient's perspective

As someone who attends specialist clinics for multiple sclerosis (MS) patients, I sometimes find that the health professionals (both doctors and nurses) lean heavily on their previous experiences with MS patients, rather than listening to my specific symptoms and my worries. The net result is that I have, on occasions, been advised, or indeed, treated for symptoms they think I should have, rather than symptoms I've actually got. This relates to previous comments about 'labels' (see Chapter 5) and certain conclusions that health professionals can wrongly (or rightly) make.

An example: for 3 years I've been prescribed medicines for bladder retention and have always queried the diagnosis (even though many MS patients do suffer from retention). After recent investigations, it has now been decided that I have an overactive bladder (no retention problem) and will shortly have a Botox injection in the bladder wall – instead of the prescribed tablets (various), which I've always said have no effect.

Moral: Because I have an MS label, it is sometimes easy for health professionals to look no further than the label, and adopt their own agenda. Perhaps this is another form of value judgment – the value needed though is again communication and exploring the patient's views of the problem.

Conclusion

While the main theme of this chapter was referral and the concept of 'ownership' of patients and professionals, we have also considered continuity, responsibility and respect: three core values for health professionals. The first of these may be difficult to maintain in the modern health service, but we can try where possible.

References

Freeman G. (1985). Priority given by doctors to continuity of care. *Journal of the Royal College of General Practitioners*, 5;423–426.

Freeman G and Hjortdahl P. (1997). What future for continuity of care in general practice? *BMJ*, **341**;1870.

General Medical Council. (2006). *Good medical practice*. London: GMC.

Haggerty JL, Reid RJ, Freeman GK, Starfield BH, Adiar CE and McKendry R. (2003). Continuity of care: a multidisciplinary review. *BMJ*, **327**;1219–1221.

Lim I. (2011). A social network approach to studying interprofessional communication. Presentation at the AMEE conference, France.

Manidis M, Slade S, McGregor J, et al. (2009). *Emergency communication: report for Prince of Wales Hospital*. Sydney: UTS.

WONCA Europe. (2002). *The European definition of general practice/family medicine*. Europe: WONCA.

13 Living with visible difference and valuing appearance

This chapter explores values in relation to appearance and the relationship between what we think about how we look and health. We consider the concept of visible difference and how we, as a society, decide on what is 'normal' (and not a health issue) and what is abnormal (and requires treatment).

Is our society concerned too much with looks? Individuals may not agree about what they value as beauty and attractiveness but most of us have a template of 'normality' that we refer to in order to distinguish difference or what we may refer to as disability or disfigurement. This chapter is in two main parts. The first is concerned with 'visible difference', a term preferred to disfigurement, which is a very value-laden concept. The second is about appearance and the possible role of health professionals when interacting with people who want to change how they look in order to improve their 'attractiveness' (as defined by the patient or client).

Reflection point

As an individual, rather than a professional, what do you consider physically attractive in another person? In our youth we may say 'I fancy X because'. While we may place a high value on intelligence, sense of humour or interpersonal skills, our initial attraction is likely to be the look of someone. How may what you consider attractive affect your professional interactions (and this could be with patients or colleagues)? Do you act differently in the presence of 'beauty'? And conversely in the absence of beauty?

Karen's story

Karen is a 24 year old machinist. When she was 4 she was badly scalded in an accident involving a pan of boiling water. She has very noticeable scarring over the right side of her face and right shoulder due to skin damage and subsequent grafting. Her right eye is distorted by damage to the upper eyelid. It is often the first thing you notice about her as she walks into the room. Karen is used to the looks and whispers about her appearance. She has found it very hard to get work in any service industry that involves direct consumer contact, though overt discrimination is hard to prove. She is shy and therefore also comes across poorly at interview. Her conclusion is that people are worried she will frighten customers, and frightened customers are unlikely to spend money.

Since she was little Karen has had the same GP, though rarely consults as she is wary and tired of medical treatment since her experience at the burns unit over the many years since her accident. She recognises her management was exemplary but so many hospital visits have made her reluctant to label herself as a patient again. Her GP is also the family doctor for her mother and younger sister and, as Karen still lives at home, when she decides she wants to go on the contraceptive pill she makes an appointment with the practice nurse Lisa Morgan, whom she has never met before. She realises that doctors are bound by the values of confidentiality, but she worries about having to enter into a polite conversation about her mother rather than concentrating on her own request. Moreover she has concerns that the GP will judge her in some way for being sexually active as he has known her since she was a baby. She is glad that she has the choice of whom to consult in her practice and is not coerced into seeing one particular professional.

What might go through Lisa's mind when Karen enters the room? Being professional means that we don't usually display our emotions in the way that perhaps the people in the waiting room do: the child who points, the young man who looks away. Perhaps the first thought is how did that happen? We may feel sorry for a young woman whose face is disfigured. We may even jump to the conclusion that she might be disabled in other ways – and in thinking that we are already labelling her as disabled purely, at this point, on the basis of her appearance.

When Karen says she would like to go on the pill, she notices that Lisa looks surprised. Why the surprise? Karen thinks it is because Lisa wonders how she has managed to get a boyfriend, whereas in fact Lisa finds it unusual for someone from Karen's estate (in a low socio-economic area) not to be on the pill already by the age of 24. We are quick to judge and such judgments occur on both sides of the office desk. Lisa carries out her usual consultation for a new pill prescription, including asking about previous medical problems. Karen does not mention the burns. Lisa is unsure whether to mention this, as there is no reason they should affect whether Karen can take the pill or not. She decides not to refer to the scarring and carries on with the consultation.

There are a number of issues here around values, which are worth exploring. The first has nothing to do with Karen's burns. Why might she be reluctant to see her usual 'family doctor' for a routine pill request? How confident are patients about the professional, and indeed ethical, value of confidentiality? Perhaps Karen is more concerned that the doctor she has seen since a child is likely to be too fatherly and judgmental about her request for contraception. She might feel embarrassed, realising that she is likely to be asked questions about her sexual history. Patients make choices about the health professionals they consult based on prior experience, wish for anonymity, gender, age and the professional's likely values.

The two main actors in this story also make value judgments about each other. Karen, who lacks confidence with new people, considers that Lisa would find her unattractive and therefore also unattractive to men. Lisa, in fact, judges Karen more in terms of her address and social standing: those girls from the estate are usually having sex at 14 and many are single mothers at 16.

Should Lisa mention Karen's scarring? Is it worse to ignore it knowing that they both know it is present (the elephant in the room)? Karen wonders how much the various health professionals at the surgery discuss each other's cases over coffee. Would her GP instantly realise who she was if Lisa mentioned she had seen a girl with dreadful facial scarring?

Reflection point

When you see a new patient or client how much information about their back story do you try to elicit? Much of this may be in their computerised records, but even then the story often needs re-interpreting. Would you enquire about Karen's appearance? What might be the advantages and disadvantages of doing so? Or the advantages and disadvantages of not doing so?

Lisa considers the consultation

When Lisa reflects on her day's consultations, she realises she knows very little about facial disfigurement and what might be done to lessen its impact. She finds a few websites about skin camouflage (Box 13.1). There is also information on the NHS website about camouflage for scarring and hyperpigmentation: http://www.nhs.uk/conditions/Scars/Pages/Introduction. aspx (Interesting use of the word camouflage here rather than make-up, what might this be saying about how we view blending in?)

Box 13.1: Skin camouflage

- Skin camouflage is the skilled application of specially formulated creams designed to minimise and neutralise defects or discolouration of the skin by covering, concealing and masking them at surface level.
- The treatment means that your appearance is improved as the focus is no longer on the defect or discolouration that you wish to hide; potentially improving your confidence and self-esteem.
- Skin camouflage techniques can be used to conceal a number of conditions, such as post-surgical concealment, scars, burns, birthmarks, rosacea, vitiligo and other pigmentation problems.
- Some camouflage creams are available through the NHS and can be prescribed by your doctor. The products can also be ordered at local pharmacies or purchased directly from the manufacturers or distributors. The prices of creams will vary according to the brand and type used. As skin colours and conditions differ it is advisable to seek professional help to find the right brand for you.'
From: http://www.consultingroom.com/Treatments/Skin-Camouflage (Accessed November 2011).

Lisa is unsure whether she should ask Karen if she is aware of camouflage creams. She didn't think that Karen was wearing anything special to hide her burns, but if she were to ask her about the problem, would Karen think she needed to mask her appearance? By drawing attention to her face would Lisa be suggesting that something needed to be done for Karen to look 'more normal'? On the other hand, perhaps Karen would be grateful for some help as it is likely that the various treatments available now are much better than they had been when she was a child. Karen might not be aware of what is on the market now and what is on prescription.

During her searching into the topic Lisa finds that many people prefer the term 'visible difference' to facial disfigurement, as the latter has more negative connotations and is very value laden. She is amazed to read the figure on the website of the charity 'Changing Faces' (http://www.changingfaces.org.uk/Home) that over one million adults and children in the UK have conditions which affect the appearance of their face or body. *Changing Faces* moreover recommends an addition to the existing multi-disciplinary teams of many health centres: 'Alongside all members of the multi-disciplinary team being trained in psycho-social care (as appropriate to their level of expertise), at *Changing Faces* we highly recommend having a psycho-social specialist integrated as part of your team. This helps to provide a clear seamless referral mechanism for patients and can help to reduce the stigma of being referred to a psychologist. However, we do realise that due to funding restrictions and staff availability and accessibility that having a dedicated psycho-social specialist on site at all times is not always a possibility' (*Changing Faces* online). Lisa does not know what training or role a psycho-social specialist has but is aware of the importance of including exploring the biopsychosocial perspective when eliciting histories from her patients. The background of this 'new' professional does appear to be psychology.

Changing Faces also includes information on 'face equality' and highlights the problems of value judgments and discrimination: 'in a culture which is increasingly obsessed with appearance and makes value judgments based on what people look like, people with disfigurements can often be rejected and treated as inferior, 'abnormal', less valuable and less able to achieve. Every day people with disfigurements face prejudice and discrimination, which can prevent them from leading happy and successful lives. They can be called names, get bullied at school, portrayed negatively in the media and can find it hard to get employment. The Face Equality campaign aims to ensure that people with disfigurements are judged fairly and treated without prejudice or discrimination' (*Changing Faces* online).

Reflection point

Consider what you feel about visible difference: have you interacted with patients with such differences? Could you see beyond it and not relate all their problems to their appearance? Should you be proactive in discussing possible management options or might this be seen as a value judgment in itself? Note the suggestion about involving yet another professional's expertise (and also consider my use of the words *yet another*). Do you think this is necessary? How would you go about finding out more about this professional's scope of practice?

Karen's consultation: a lay perspective

The following is written by a colleague and friend who had traumatic injuries to her face as a child.

As a woman who has lived with visible difference for most of her life, I empathise with the situation that Karen quite literally faces, having experienced similar scenarios myself. However, though I share the experience of living with 'disfigurement', it's important to remember that each individual's response to disfigurement will be different; indeed research has shown that there is no relation between the severity of the disfigurement and the level of distress arising from it. The assumption cannot be made that Karen's apparent lack of confidence is due to her scarring; this could have arisen for a variety of reasons.

Karen's need for contraception reminded me just how much I hated consulting my GP about matters relating to birth control. As in the scenario above, the male GP was the family doctor and I was concerned that he would tell my mother, so I asked for 'The Pill' because friends had told me what great relief it provided for menstrual cramps when everything else had failed. Thereafter I discovered that I could get contraception from the family planning clinic, without having to justify myself and unbeknown to my parents!

I did find it disquieting that the nurse, Lisa, even thought about asking about Karen's burns, although experience has taught me that this is not an untypical response. Health care professionals are prone to make comments like 'what an interesting scar that is' – interesting to whom? And just what is that comment meant to add to the consultation? However the nurse may appraise Karen, the burns are unlikely to be relevant to her request for contraception since any underlying/disabling medical condition would surely come to light during the routine health assessment prior to contraception being prescribed.

I do question how likely it is that health care professionals confuse disfigurement with disability particularly when the disfigurement is facial and the patient walks unaided into the consultation room. However, such confusion – if it exists – is understandable given that disfigurement and disability are treated alike in the UK's Disability and Equality Act 2010, which unhelpfully states that a person has a disability if 'they have a physical or mental impairment'.

Karen, who apparently lacks confidence with new people, may well attribute Lisa's surprise at her request for contraception to her own lack of self-esteem; but this is questionable. Karen clearly has acquired a boyfriend, which suggests that her social skills are more than adequate, even though developing intimate relationships may be challenging to people living with disfigurement. It's all too easy to make assumptions about how a disfigurement will be perceived by others, in this case by men. Some men will be put off by disfigurement others will not. Quite frankly I didn't give a thought as to whether or not I would attract a boyfriend. That never occurred to me, I was just scared witless about falling pregnant! We are all in danger of imposing one's own standards and prejudices on others, I'm conscious I do it all the time.

In this story Lisa, in fact, judges Karen more in terms of her postcode and social standing, her surprise relating to the fact that someone of Karen's age has not requested contraception earlier. The nurse might have put Karen more at ease had she complimented her on her decision to seek contraceptive advice when so many local young people failed to do so.

In some respects I don't think the scarring is pertinent to this discussion unless it involves an underlying medical condition. If both parties know there's an elephant in the room why comment on it? If Karen feels uncomfortable with her scarring she will find some way of letting the health care professional know even though she is shy. The fact that Karen is even thinking about the need for contraception kind of suggests she's not that shy…but in fact anticipates an intimate relationship and is acting responsibly to avoid an unwanted pregnancy.

On the other hand, if the nurse hasn't met Karen before, Karen might want to satisfy the nurse's unspoken curiosity – something I often do. I know when people want to ask me about my scar but are too polite to do so, or cannot find a suitable way of expressing their curiosity. Sometimes a quick explanation can overcome those unspoken questions and provide the health care professional (and others!) with an opportunity to ask if there are any ongoing problems or treatments. For example, the burns may get dry and sore from time to time and require a lubricant! Whatever, the topic can be laid to rest and everyone can move on.

Reflection point

Did anything surprise you about the above patient interlude? Will you do anything different as a result?

More discussion about appearance

On the first Wednesday afternoon of every month Darpington Surgery has a 3 hour protected professional development session. All the members of the primary health care team working out of the health centre are invited to attend. This afternoon Jessica Parry, one of the two nurse practitioners, has suggested the topic of 'appearance', a title that intrigued the other staff members. The content was illuminated when Jessica asked each health professional to be ready to discuss a patient or client who was concerned about or disliked his or her looks such as size, shape, scarring or disfigurement etc.

Jessica leads the session. In attendance are five GPs (three male and two female) with variable experience, a GP registrar, her fellow nurse practitioner (Tom), three practice nurses, a practice counselor, a physiotherapist and the practice manager (William). She begins by asking all present to say what they like and dislike about their own appearance and, that at this point, no-one is to comment on what the others are saying. To give them time to think Jessica says she likes her eyes but thinks her thighs are too big. The likes of the team include hair, feet, smile and eyelashes; the dislikes are mainly related to shape and size: bottom, calves, upper arms (bingo wings as nurse Debbie says) and general flab (William). Tom also says 'bald patch' and Maggie (52 year old GP) wrinkles round her mouth and eyes.

Jessica then asks: 'Now how many of you would consult a health professional about any of your dislikes?' This question causes some amusement and also some embarrassed looks. Tom admits to seeing his GP a few years ago about his bald patch, was reassured it was normal male pattern balding and not medical alopecia and then went to a private clinic to discuss hair restoration treatment. 'Too expensive in the end and anyway my girlfriend said we should spend the money on our honeymoon instead.' He grins. 'She values a 5 star hotel over my looks.' Maggie surprises the group by saying she has recently considered Botox or facial fillers to rejuvenate her looks, but then decided she was being silly and who did she have to impress but herself. In the end she says she valued her health (and her bank balance) more than her features, but that she can understand why other women might want to have injections or plastic surgery.

Though a few people want to respond to Maggie, Jessica moves them on. 'That was to show that no-one is ever fully satisfied with how they look; but for some people appearance is more important than for others. We might think their concerns are trivial. Can we empathise with patients who want to alter their looks?'

Jessica tells about a recent consultation, which precipitated her wish to discuss appearance at this meeting (Box 13.2).

Box 13.2: Kate and her breasts

'Kate is a 20 year old supermarket cashier who came in to talk about her breast size. She is a 36 EE and is very unhappy with her shape. She gets back pain and would like to do more exercise but finds it very hard to get a bra to fit to do any sort of jogging. What makes it worse for her is that many of her friends are envious of her cleavage and can't understand what the problem is. They say that blokes love big boobs and one of them is even trying to save up to have breast implants. She hasn't got a boyfriend at the moment, but certainly her last one loved her breasts which is why she hasn't been in to see anyone so far. She wanted to see a female nurse I presume because she thought I would be more sympathetic. She is a bit overweight but certainly her breasts are out of proportion to her general shape'.

There is a discussion about whether this is a health problem for Kate and the consensus is that it probably is. Breast reductions can be done on the NHS (without charge) as long as the breasts are impairing a person's life but the question then arises as to what size Kate would want her 'new' breasts to be. The only dissenting opinion is Peter, the oldest GP present at 63. He feels that in these days of health spending cuts that breast reduction, which is after all about appearance, is not a priority. 'If young women are prepared to save to get their breasts larger, then they can also save to get them smaller.' Jessica asks whether Kate's referral should depend on the values of the consulting professional, or whether there should be a standard that everyone adheres to. 'I have advised her to see a female GP for a referral. Good job I didn't recommend you Peter. Is it fair that a personal opinion affects referral or treatment? Even a personal value in good faith based on health economics and the state of the health service?'

Is breast reduction in these circumstances similar to liposuction (a privately funded procedure) or gastric banding (which can now be carried out by health service funding in some areas if a patient is morbidly obese)? The group considers that the outcome is dependent on the health status of the patient and whether the operation is to improve health and reduce morbidity, or to improve appearance without health benefits. However psychological benefits are hard to measure in such cases. Tom suggests that hair transplants will never be considered for public funding even if a man's confidence would be helped. 'It's just something that you have to accept as your genetic lot in life.'

Mairead, the counselor, sees a lot of clients with body issues – they can lead to lack of confidence and sometimes depression. However there are often other underlying problems besides the hated physical features. Treatment of these may help to resolve the body issues or at least facilitate clients to consider ways of coping with or ameliorating the condition. Mairead goes onto say that the problem for the other health professionals is lack of time within a consultation to explore a client's ideas and values. She has the luxury of 30–60 minute appointments, but only for six sessions 'which is often not enough'.

The GP registrar, Colin, wonders how much a doctor should know about beauty treatments which are outside mainstream medicine, such as aesthetic plastic surgery and medication for skin whitening for example. 'I have been asked in the last few weeks about my opinions on facial fillers, silicon implants and tattoo removal, even penis enlargement, none of which I know much about. And it isn't just about the safety and risk aspects, some patients want my actual opinions – do you think I should have it done doctor?' Maggie suggests this is because Colin is younger than most of the rest of the team and is probably thought by some of the patients to be more aware of what could be called fashion trends. 'I read the other day that there are even procedures now to increase the size of the buttocks, yet other women are afraid that their bums might look too big. I don't always understand you women at all' Peter says (ignoring the topic of penile implants).

There is general agreement that a sub-set of the 'younger' generation values attractiveness above other attributes such as intelligence and physical fitness. Examples suggesting this are given as young women smoking to stay thin and the use of sun beds for that 'attractive tan'. Jessica suggests that as health professionals they need to be non-judgmental about these patient values, listen to what the patient is asking, give unbiased facts, warn against obviously dangerous behaviour, but otherwise give the patient space to make up their own mind. This is obviously easier if there is no question of NHS referral for treatment; once a professional moves into the gatekeeping role in terms of deciding who to refer for breast reduction or treatment for acne scarring, for example, the values of the professional are more likely to be important. A referral might not always lead to treatment if the hospital specialist disagrees; the specialist also operates with values: his/her own plus that of the hospital board. However the referral and subsequent out-patient appointment do take up time and cost money.

Colin says he finds it hard to be objective when women complain of imperfections that to him seem perfectly normal. 'There is such peer pressure to conform. Sometimes I think that people have lost the sense of the diversity of normality, don't really know what is abnormal and are chasing an ideal version of someone else's opinions publicised through the media.' While a certain treatment might not be available through the NHS and public funding, if people are prepared to pay, then a doctor will be prepared to operate. Are therapeutic decisions made differently if a direct fee is involved? Can, and should, money buy you everything?

While there may be a health system policy on who can be referred for cosmetic surgery for example, the practice may also decide to have its own policy. Of course 'the practice' is made up of individual team members, with their values and experience. How is the policy decided? By democratic vote or the power of the leadership, which is likely to be the doctors? A policy may be decided by the majority but the dissenters will then have to work within this policy even though it disagrees with their values. Corporate values are thus important as a source of possible conflict.

Appearance and values

One of the benefits of these practice education meetings is the chance for the health professionals to discuss difficult cases, get advice from colleagues and ratify their decisions. Ruth, a 38 year old GP, wants to talk about obesity and dealing with overweight patients. She used to have a BMI of 30 herself but over the last year has lost several stones (kilograms) through a combination of careful eating and exercise.

'I am really struggling with this issue at the moment. I attract patients who want to change their body shape, probably because they have seen what I have managed. The patients who realise it is going to be a hard slog are fine; they mainly need advice, motivation and encouragement. Many of them are happy to come to the support group run by Ann (practice nurse) and Janice (physiotherapist, who discusses exercise regimens taking into consideration the patient's underlying health). But there are two types of patient whom I find difficult to interact with. The first are the patients who want to lose weight but think there is a tablet that will do all the hard work for them, those wonderful slimming tablets just to kick start their metabolism. For these patients the problem is anyone's fault but their own: their glands, their metabolism, their lack of time, the price of food etc. They think that I am withholding treatment from them that I had access to as a doctor. I get so frustrated. The other group is the patients who are unhappy with a certain feature of their appearance and want to spot reduce their thighs, or bums or tums. I'm not sure why they think this is a medical problem with a medical solution, except that we are a 'free' service compared to the gym and personal trainers. I try the usual things about looking for underlying agendas or concerns, but they just seem to think that it is their right and it is possible to look like J-Lo or Beyonce.'

One hallmark of our modern Western society is that a large section of the population appears to be obsessed with the way they look. We see this manifested as a concern about weight and an obsession to be thin (the size zero phenomenon), about ageing and the desire to continue to look young (Botox and plastic surgery) and about breast and bottom size (too big, too small, not perfect). Some commentators feel that these obsessions are fuelled by the cult of celebrity and aspirations to look perfect. We become more critical of ourselves and others if we do not match some pre-defined image of beauty. Of course, this definition changes according to trends and is manipulated by commercial interests selling new products to reduce weight, combat ageing, change skin colour and remove impurities.

Many of us do value looking good, though we may define 'good' in different ways. There are potential clashes of values in the health care field when someone (usually the organisation controlling health care spending) decides whether treatment to correct body imperfections or disfigurement is fundable through the public health care system. So, for example, bat ears in children may be paid for by the NHS but a crooked nose may not (unless it affects breathing). Moreover such decisions are not always the same in different parts of the country: the so called health care lottery or postcode rationing. These decisions are often based on values rather than evidence. Unless there are physical reasons for surgery or other treatments (as in the case of the nose), a patient has to have psychological problems or the potential for psychological harm in order to have such management agreed. The power of the referring professional and fund holder (via commissioning) is immense. What might seem a trivial request to them, could be an overwhelming issue to a patient without clinical evidence of mental health problems. The scar on someone's face to one person is tiny; to another it is huge.

Research has shown that familial values are important in how adolescent girls in particular view their weight and appearance, and that these values differ across social classes (Ogden & Thomas, 1999). Girls from more affluent families (at fee paying schools for instance) were found to be more concerned about their weight and had greater levels of dissatisfaction with their figures while being more restrained in their eating habits, compared to teenagers in state comprehensive schools. The evidence base around values in obesity has been explored by Petrova and her colleagues (Petrova et al., 2006).

Pitfalls of appearance

How much do our own criteria of what looks good and what looks normal affect our interactions with patients, and indeed with our colleagues? Our feelings can be very complex. I might consider an obese female patient to have let herself go, to have no will power, to be over indulgent, precisely because that is very different to the way I live. But if a colleague loses weight and begins to get compliments for her new look and her efforts, do I feel envious and threatened? Weight maintenance and loss can become almost a competition, an outward expression of the value placed on body proportions. Telling someone 'you have lost weight' can mean, or be interpreted to mean:

- Well done for losing weight.
- Wow, you look really good now.
- You were too big before.
- Are you ill?
- I am concerned about you.

What a professional may say in a consultation is different from what we might say in civilian life. A long time dieter, someone who finds it hard to keep slim, becomes very frustrated at a patient who wants to put on weight. There is the girl who 'no matter what I eat I can't seem to gain weight' who makes us very envious, the woman who wants to exercise to enlarge her breasts but otherwise stay the same size; the man who wants muscles and is obviously taking steroids but denies it. It is important to be able to pick up the patients with the eating disorders (Box 13.3) – when does a weight obsession become a mental health problem? The other condition linked to appearance is body dysmorphic disorder (BDD), which is a serious illness and manifests as a person being obsessed with minor or imaginary physical flaws, usually of the skin, hair and nose. Could our own values blind us to real mental distress?

Box 13.3: Eating disorders (from the Mayo Clinic online)

- Eating disorders are a group of serious conditions in which you're so preoccupied with food and weight that you can often focus on little else. The main types of eating disorders are anorexia nervosa, bulimia nervosa and binge-eating disorder.
- Eating disorders can cause serious physical problems and at their most severe can even be life-threatening. Most people with eating disorders are females, but males can also have eating disorders. An exception is binge-eating disorder, which appears to affect almost as many males as females.
- Treatments for eating disorders usually involve psychotherapy, nutrition education, family counselling, medications and hospitalisation.

Conclusion

We do live in a part of the world where appearance to many is very important. There is sometimes a fine line between a health problem and a social problem, or what some may say is no problem at all. As with other topics there is likely to be a difference between the personal and professional values of team members and the values of our patients and clients. Discussion about appearance may be very exasperating if we find the patient's value trivial or resistant to change. By discussing our values with colleagues we may gain a greater insight into diversity and how we may collaborate to improve patient care.

References

Mayo Clinic online. (2011). Available at: www.mayoclinic.com/health/eating-disorders/DS00294 (Accessed November 2011).

Ogden J and Thomas D. (1999). The role of familial values in understanding the impact of social class on weight concern. *International Journal of Eating Disorders*, 25;273–279.

Petrova M, Dale J and Fulford B. (2006) Values-based practice in primary care: easing the tensions between individual values, ethical principles and best evidence. *British Journal of General Practice*, 56;703–709.

14

Collaboration with other professionals: in and outside health care

There are a number of professionals who are not regular members of the health care team, or who are not health professionals themselves, but who are vitally important for optimal and safe patient care. Often these are the professionals whose roles are poorly understood and whose full repertoire of skills is under-utilised. In this chapter we explore the role of some of these: specifically the pharmacist, the teacher, the police officer and the social worker.

> **Reflection point**
>
> Which of these professionals would you recognise as part of your team – possibly a temporary member? Think of interactions with any of these people: what went well and why; what could have been done differently to improve the situation. Do you have a good understanding of their scope of practice? What do you immediately think of if asked to suggest their values?

Alan the pharmacist

Alan Goodacre has recently taken over the running of the local pharmacy. The shop is part of a large national franchise and sells the usual cosmetics and toiletries as well as over the counter (OTC) medication. Alan qualified 10 years ago and has worked in both hospital and community settings since he received his degree. He is keen to establish a good working relationship with the general practices whose patients come to him for their medicine to be dispensed. In the last few weeks he has made appointments with the practice managers and some of the doctors at several clinics. Some have made him feel very welcome, while others have appeared rushed and almost rude.

One evening Julie Sellars comes into the shop and asks to speak to the 'chemist'. She says she wants the morning after pill. Alan has a quiet corner behind at the end of the counter where he can discuss confidential information with customers so as not to be overheard by anyone else on the premises. His assistant deals with other people while he attends to Julie's request. He finds out that Julie is 19, that she had an accident with a split condom the previous evening, that she is healthy and has only used emergency contraception (the preferred terminology) once before about 2 years ago. Alan is happy to dispense the necessary pill but advises Julie that as she has no prescription there will be a charge for the treatment. Julie is a little tearful and says she has tried to get an appointment at her GP surgery but there is nothing available for two days. She had told the receptionist it was urgent but didn't want to say what the problem was over the phone as it was no business of hers. The cost is a surprise as she thought that all contraception was free. She will have to pay with her credit card.

Alan checks the pharmacy database but has no record for Julie. He gives her the pill and suggests that she may want to consider a more effective method of contraception than condoms in the future. He advises her to discuss contraception with someone at the practice in the next few weeks and also what to do if her period is late. (What Julie hasn't told Alan is that the 'morning after pill' is her preferred method of contraception and that in fact she has had three prescriptions in the last 6 months: one from her own practice and two from different walk-in centres in the town – all free of charge. She doesn't want another 'lecture' on why this lifestyle is not recommended. She had tried to see the practice nurse rather than a doctor as she thinks nurses are a softer touch; but even the nurse was full.)

An hour later, just before he closes for the night, Alan is handed a prescription for erythromycin (commonly prescribed antibiotic particularly for patients allergic to penicillin) in the name of Zayn Rajgupta. Alan checks his computer noting that Zayn is also on several other medications for heart disease including a statin (cholesterol lowering agent). Erythromycin and this statin should not be taken together due to the risk of side effects. The prescription is from the same practice where Julie was unable to see a doctor or nurse that evening. Alan rings the surgery and asks to speak to the responsible GP, stating who he is and that he has a query about a patient's prescription. After waiting for a few minutes the receptionist tells him that the doctor is busy and cannot take his call and that Alan should ring back in the morning. Alan insists he needs to discuss the problem now and therefore the doctor should call him when free. But there is no return call in the next 20 minutes, and when Alan tries the number again (15 minutes after his closing time), he hears a message that the surgery is now shut and that for urgent problems patients are advised to contact the out of hours service. Later that week Alan has an appointment at Mr Rajgupta's practice.

Reflection point

What are your feelings in relation to this scenario and how are these affected by your profession, your values and your experiences? How may pharmacists work with practice-based health professionals and what impact may this have on patient care?

Different professions – different values?

We have considered this aspect of teamwork several times in this book, with the underlying message that team members need to discuss their personal and professional values to improve collaboration, communication and patient care. But how may we do this if we are really not a team? Alan and the primary care teams with which he interacts because of 'shared' patients do not meet regularly, do not discuss the patient's goals and agree on the management plan and do not consider how they may improve the way they work. These are the objectives for 'true' teams that were defined in Chapter 2, page 68.

When I reflect on my own medical training I always remember that I had no idea there was such a person as a 'hospital pharmacist' until my first year working as a qualified junior doctor. As a student I had never been shown round the hospital pharmacy or seen how the drugs that I would prescribe on the wards were checked or dispensed. As a GP in training (GP registrar) I was timetabled to spend half a day at the local community pharmacy (also known as the chemist's shop) and saw what happened to prescriptions and the questions that patients asked the pharmacist (presumably that they hadn't thought to or been comfortable to ask their GP). These days health professional students who undertake some form of interprofessional education meet and learn with pharmacy students to dispel some of the myths about each other.

Alan is keen to have better links with his local prescribers. He likes to be able to put a face to a name and a voice if he has to ring a practice because of queries about prescriptions. He assumes that the GPs and nurses will also feel more comfortable talking to him and taking advice if they have met him and have some understanding of his values. Let's consider what the actors in the above scenario think about each other's roles and values and how these thoughts compare with what they think about themselves (Box 14.1). While these are obviously speculations, what is interesting is that health professionals who do rarely meet and whose interactions are through their patients-in-common may have very little understanding of each other's values. Even though misunderstanding is also possible within teams, the chances of this occurring are much more likely between professionals such as Alan and the GP in the scenario who have never met. Their assumptions about each other's attitudes to patient care are based on hearsay and through the actions of the receptionist go-between, plus their previous experiences of working with pharmacists/GPs in the past.

But there is published evidence to suggest that the some of the speculation in Box 14.1 is likely to be close to the truth. A qualitative study of GPs and community pharmacists in Northern Ireland, published in 2003, highlighted a number of barriers to effective collaboration between the two professions. While based on small numbers of interviewees, the results resonate with other research in this area. The GPs felt that pharmacists would have conflicts between their 'shopkeeper' position and their role in health care, while the pharmacists reported difficulty in accessing the GPs because of the behaviour of the doctors' receptionists. The pharmacists also considered that GPs had little understanding and appreciation of their role (Hughes and McCann, 2003).

I was involved in a small pilot educational project at one university in which we involved pharmacy and medical students undertaking a medicine review for a simulated patient (for more on working with simulated patients see Chapter 15). The students worked in pairs to interview the patient and then make decisions about rationalising her prescriptions. For the evaluation of the project we asked the students for their views on each other's way of working and what they had learnt about their peers. The pharmacy students said they now realised that medical students were more caring than they had previously believed (usually before meeting any) and that they communicated very well with the patient, exploring more about the patient's social circumstances and ideas than the pharmacy students did. The medical students were very impressed by the knowledge of medicines and interactions that the pharmacy students had at this stage of their training and realised that pharmacists would be very helpful colleagues in the future (Ajjawi et al., 2010).

While doctors and nurses with prescribing rights may consider that pharmacists are mainly out to make a profit, involving pharmacists more in medication review and consultations with patients on multiple drugs is about patient safety (less confusion with dosages) and cost saving to the health service. Pharmacists have a better knowledge of the cost of drugs, can suggest cheaper but as effective alternatives, may rationalise the number of times a medication has to be taken daily (for example changing from a three times a day dose to a once a day formulation) and provide dosette boxes to help the elderly adhere to their drug regimens. Some general practices now employ a pharmacist for a session or more a week to advise on prescribing and to help keep doctors and nurses up-to-date in relation to medicines.

Box 14.1: Professional and personal values

	Alan	GP	Receptionist	Julie	Mr Rajgupta
Alan	Values his patients as customers – but puts their well-being over profit. He does sell OTC medication and other remedies for which there is patchy evidence but which the patients want. Tends to believe what patients tell him (such as Julie) though thinks he has good intuition to pick up drug seekers and addicts. He enjoys interacting with patients/ customers and thinks that pharmacists' knowledge and skills are under used in most cases.	Alan has great respect for most doctors but they have to earn it. He feels some make a lot of money without providing good care. He has put a black mark against Mr Rajgupta's GP for not only prescribing poorly (not checking a drug interaction) but also not having professional courtesy to answer his call.	Alan feels that when he rings a GP he should be put straight through and not have to wait or be put on hold by a receptionist. Sometimes he thinks that receptionists have too much power over other professionals and the patients.	Has no reason to doubt what Julie is saying to him. Feels sorry for her that she could not get a free prescription from her practice but he is not prepared to give her the pill without charge – he has the right to charge and needs to make a profit.	Even though Alan is annoyed with the GP, his professional values at this point mean that he will not make disparaging remarks about the doctor to his patient.
GP	This GP has little to do with pharmacists. He rarely meets one professionally. He feels that pharmacists are shop keepers (with customers rather than patients), eager to make money out of sick people and that they sell anything to anyone including 'worthless' homeopathic remedies. He does get rung up if there are	This GP does not like being interrupted during consultations, as he likes to give patients his undivided attention. He does not always check his messages at the end of the day, or fit in 'extras' unless real emergencies as he likes to get home to his family.	He expects the receptionist to make his life comfortable and sort out problems so he can be left to do what he is good at: healing patients.	Does not consider the need for emergency contraception as an emergency as there are plenty of other places to get the pill. He would tell Julie off for relying on this method – she should be using a long acting injection or implant to avoid becoming a single mum – or better still avoid having sex altogether.	OK – he has made a mistake and can sort it out tomorrow – the antibiotics are not urgent for tonight. He will apologise to the patient next time he sees him. The computer must have been at fault in not picking up the interaction or it is so rare as to be unimportant (except to a pharmacist).

Box 14.1: (cont.)

	Alan	GP	Receptionist	Julie	Mr Rajgupta
	problems with prescriptions and sometimes feels that as pharmacists do want more autonomy, they should make more decisions on their own instead of bothering him.				
Receptionist	A pharmacist is an important professional but this GP will be annoyed if she interrupts him. The GP comes before the pharmacist.	The doctor is fine if she does not overload him with either problems or patients.	Does her job well. Puts the happiness of the doctors before the patients. Some patients try it on to get an appointment but she knows when things are serious.	Julie wouldn't state her problem so can't be urgent and she can wait until there is a free slot. Some of these young girls are so demanding and need everything now.	A lovely man. Always polite and happy to wait his turn.
Julie	Should the pharmacist be charging her for this? What a price? He seems ok but he is not a doctor – why is he asking her all these questions. She will just bend the truth to avoid too much probing.	Why don't the doctors like giving out emergency contraception as a method? It means you don't have to take pills all the time. Bet this doctor would prefer no-one to have sex or fun.	'A dragon! Why should I tell her what's wrong?'	'I'm being responsible by asking for the morning after pill – they would soon complain if I wanted an abortion.'	
Mr Rajgupta	Doesn't ask pharmacists for advice as usually his own doctor is very informative. 'Why won't he give me my pills?'	'Lovely man, always takes time with you.' Has great respect for doctors.	And their receptionists.		Doesn't expect doctors to make mistakes – very trusting and tends not to ask questions

A Cochrane review of the effects of integration of pharmacists into primary care teams suggested that this intervention enhances the quality of prescribing and improves patient outcomes, though the studies in this area did tend to be of poor quality (Bero et al., 2000). Moreover pharmacists have been shown to increase the effectiveness of team interventions in the management of chronic illness in the community (Wagner, 2006). In hospitals, the participation of pharmacists on ward rounds with other medical and nursing staff has long been shown to reduce the number of adverse events relating to prescribed medication, as well as reducing drug costs (Leape et al., 1999). This collaboration generally leads to improvement in patient care and includes pharmacists counselling patients about their medication before discharge from hospital (Kaboli et al., 2006). By encouraging more interaction between the professionals such initiatives build respect and are likely to indicate that there is a great deal of overlap between our values in relation to health care delivery.

Reflection point

If you are not a pharmacist, how much do you know about this profession's training and scope of practice? What do you think of when you hear the word pharmacist? How might it improve how you care for patients if you had a better relationship with your local pharmacist? Alan is going to a meeting at Julie's and Mr Rajgupta's general practice. What might be on his agenda to discuss and how does this relate to values-based practice?

The police officer, the social worker and the teacher

Each of these professions advertises a set of values (or a code of ethics in the case of social work), using similar words and concepts (Box 14.2). The wording is similar across professions, which is not surprising and there is a strong sense of public duty. We could therefore expect that these professions would work well together with a common purpose and goals. But as we have seen even health care professionals have conflicts of values, and words such as *partnership*, *empowerment* and *policing* are open to interpretation, both by professionals and the public.

A common scenario involving this trio of people, plus a health professional, is an incident of child abuse in a school age child. There are legal requirements in relation to behaviour, reporting and intervention if any professional suspects child abuse or a child confides such abuse to a teacher or other adult. Health professionals become involved in checking the child for signs of physical and/or psychological damage. The resulting inquiry usually results in a multi-disciplinary case conference. There are of course other situations where health professionals may become involved with the police, social services or the education provider. For many health professionals these may be uncommon interactions and some may be unsure of issues relating to confidentiality, disclosure and duty of care. As health professionals we may have conscious or unconscious prejudices against the police and social services, based on our values and what we assume are theirs. Many events described in great detail in the media about the failure of professionals to protect young children have led to reduced confidence in social workers and indeed doctors. We have seen people trying to pass the blame on: I did what I could, it was his/her fault for not passing on information/realising the severity of the injuries/reading the medical records/putting the child back in the family home/not putting the child back with the parents/ignoring the concerns of the neighbours etc. Such episodes

Box 14.2: Values of social work, the police and education

Profession	Values
Social work	**Human dignity and worth** Respect for human dignity and for individual and cultural diversity. Value for every human being, their beliefs, goals, preferences and needs. Respect for human rights and self-determination. Partnership and empowerment with users of services and with carers. Ensuring protection for vulnerable people. **Social justice** Promoting fair access to resources. Equal treatment without prejudice or discrimination. Reducing disadvantage and exclusion. Challenging the abuse of power. **Service** Helping with personal and social needs. Enabling people to develop their potential. Contributing to the creation of a fairer society. **Integrity** Honesty, reliability and confidentiality. **Competence** Maintaining and expanding competence to provide a quality service. Available from: www.basw.co.uk/about/code-of-ethics/ (accessed January 2012).
Police	Working together with all our citizens, all our partners, all our colleagues: • We will have pride in delivering quality policing. There is no greater priority. • We will build trust by listening and responding. • We will respect and support each other and work as a team. • We will learn from experience and find ways to be even better. Note: this is from the Metropolitan Police Force (London).
Education	Value and demonstrate a commitment to social justice, inclusion and protecting and caring for children. Value themselves as growing professionals by taking responsibility for their professional learning and development. Value, respect and show commitment to the communities in which they work. Available from: www.gtcs.org.uk/standards/standard-initial-teacher-education.aspx (accessed January 2012).

do little for the credibility and professionalism of those concerned; the media also stir things up by looking for scapegoats and wanting to hold those involved to account.

Lay people have different expectations and feelings about these other services. For some families 'calling in the social worker' is seen as a threat and the police are always enemies rather than assistance. These ideas are often independent of whether there is something to hide or a genuine reason for concern. As professionals we may have conflicts of interest and conflicts of values: wanting to do the best for our patients but realising that we also have to balance this against the good of the community. GMC guidance, for example, is that doctors should report gunshot wounds and knife injuries to the police, even disclosing the patient's name without consent, if they consider that a serious crime has taken place or other people are at risk. In cases where we are not sure about our responsibilities and what we can or cannot disclose to other agencies, our indemnity organisation or professional bodies are able to offer advice.

A major cause of the failings within child protection is a lack of understanding by those involved of professional roles and responsibilities. For example in the case of Victoria Climbié, an 8 year old girl from the Ivory Coast who moved to the UK in 1999 to be looked after by her aunt and who died as a result of frequent physical abuse, social services and the police both thought the other agency was taking the lead on the case. Lord Laming's report on the subsequent public inquiry highlighted the confusion around responsibilities and the lack of training of some personnel for cases of this kind (Laming, 2003). As noted by Kennison & Fletcher (2005): 'For effective interprofessional working, a combination of personal and professional confidence, together with competent communication skills are required to enable individuals to challenge the views of other professionals' (p. 127). Perhaps if we value another profession too highly, we are unlikely to challenge in this way?

Twenty-four hour care and accessibility

Reflection point

If a person has an 'emergency' in the middle of the night who is available to call and who is likely to respond? What does your answer indicate about your profession's values?

In the past 'patients' in many parts of the country would have been able to ring their own doctor, or their own general practice, for help with medical problems. Now they are more likely to ring '999' in the UK (or equivalent elsewhere): the police are the only 24-hour service who may respond to any situation. If the person is able to discriminate between a medical problem and other issue, they may ask for the ambulance service (or fire service for an obvious fire) but everything else is directed to the police service. Some of these calls for help may be considered health related or have health-related repercussions, for example unexpected deaths, mental health problems involving violent or aggressive behaviour, domestic violence and road traffic accidents. There is, of course, major abuse of the 999 call service, which is regularly reported in the media. It is easy as a person with a broad and extensive education to judge these callers as time wasters but we do not know their full stories and their motivation for picking up the phone. One issue is that while mobile phones are ubiquitous and 999 calls are free, many people do not know who else to turn to for advice, because of poor social networks, and are often lacking in common sense due to poor parenting, lack of role models or mental health problems. We know that some patients come to our health centres because they are lonely and mainly want to have a conversation with a good listener. Is it our duty as professionals to be accessible for the less fortunate? Health professionals and the police sometimes feel that they are substituting for social workers, without the necessary skills and training. Unfortunately problems are not easy to put into boxes: social, health, crime...We need some overlap in our capabilities but we also need our colleagues and collaborations to provide optimum care.

Conclusion

Health care overlaps with social care, and patients are often involved with other agencies such as the police, the probation service, legal system and such services as victim support and self-help groups. Collaborative working may help in some cases; in other cases patients may prefer their professionals and problems to be separate. However this may not always be possible as the patient's wants may run counter to professional values in such areas as child protection and violent crime, and indeed what patients ask may be illegal in some cases.

References

Ajjawi R, Thistlethwaite J, Williams KA, Ryan G, Seale JP and Carroll PR. (2010). Breaking down professional barriers: medicine and pharmacy students learning together. *Focus on health professional education: A Multi-disciplinary Journal*, **12**; 1–10.

Bero LA, Mays NB, Barjesteh K and Bond C. (2000). Abstract of review: expanding outpatient pharmacists' roles and health services utilisation, costs, and patient outcomes. *Cochrane Collaboration. Cochrane Library*. Issue 1. Oxford: Update Software.

Hughes CM and McCann S. (2003). Perceived interprofessional barriers between community pharmacists and general practitioners: a qualitative study. *British Journal of General Practice*, **53**;600–606.

Kaboli PJ, Hoth AB, McCLomon BJ and Schnipper JL. (2006). Clinical pharmacists and inpatient medical care. *Annals of Internal Medicine*, **166**;955–964.

Kennison P and Fletcher R. (2005). Police. In: Barrett G, Sellman D and Thomas J (Eds). *Interprofessional working in health and social care*. Basingstoke: Palgrave Macmillan. p119–131.

Laming WH. (2003). *Inquiry into the death of Victoria Climbié*. London: The Stationery Office.

Leape LL, Cullen DJ, Clapp MD, et al. (1999). Pharmacist participation on physician rounds and adverse drug event in the intensive care unit. *Journal of the American Medical Association*, **282**;267–270.

Wagner EH. (2006). The role of patient care teams in chronic disease management. *BMJ*, **302**;569–572.

Learning in and about teams

This chapter focuses more specifically on how teams can learn to work together and education that facilitates developing skills for collaboration. In particular I discuss the concept and context of interprofessional education (IPE) and its role in understanding and working together within a values-based framework. There are two examples of interprofessional learning activities for practice teams.

Reflection point

Consider what you already know about IPE. Do you know of any definitions of IPE? In your own career how have you learnt the theory behind and skills for teamwork? Did this learning ever include outcomes relating to values-based practice?

One of the perplexing features of contemporary health care professional education, both before and after qualification, is that there is still comparatively little learning in and about teams, teamwork and collaborative practice. This is in spite of the growing awareness of the need for and development of teamwork in health care. Skills for teamwork, leadership and collaborative practice do now appear as core competencies in many health professional curricula. Some of the learning to achieve these outcomes does take place in groups and teams; some of the learning is multiprofessional and some interprofessional (Box 15.1), but summative (endpoint) assessment for qualification or registration is always of the individual. In my experience, rarely is there specific mention of values in current health professional education: individual, team, organisation or values-based practice.

Your own education

Depending on your age, experience and the year you qualified, you will have had none, some, or a great deal of interprofessional education through interprofessional learning (IPL) or more likely multiprofessional (Box 15.1). If you have experience of IPE, consider when this happened, with whom you were learning, what the intended outcomes of the learning were and whether these were achieved. Did you enjoy the activities? What would you have changed about the session/programme/workshop etc, if you were going to participate again or even run a session yourself? Has there been any other time when team work was a specific learning outcome in your education or continuing professional development (CPD) activities? How have you developed your ability to work in or lead a team? Were values ever mentioned in an educational activity?

Box 15.1: Definition of IPE and IPL

- Interprofessional education (IPE): The definition that is now commonly used internationally is that of the Centre for the Advancement of Interprofessional Education (CAIPE). The 2002 version states that IPE occurs: 'when two or more professions learn from, with and about each other to improve collaboration and the quality of care' (CAIPE, 2002). 'Professions' usually refers to health and social care, but can include other professions that collaborate to improve health and well-being such as education and law. The learners within the professions may be pre-qualification students and/or qualified practitioners. The prepositions 'from, with and about' are important as they imply that learning is shared, interactive and equitable, rather than just in common and passive. Interprofessional may be contrasted with multiprofessional education, which involves the professions learning side by side without interaction (also known as common learning).
- Interprofessional learning (IPL) or shared learning: Learning arising from interaction between members (or students) of two or more professions. This may be a product of interprofessional education or happen spontaneously in the workplace or in education settings (Freeth et al., 2005).
- In contrast multiprofessional learning (or common learning): the learners from two or more professions learn together without planned interaction to cover a common topic.

Your own experience of learning will certainly colour your recommendations to others about how they should learn. But some of the most powerful influences on your subsequent working practice will have been the people you learnt with, from and observed in the clinical environment. As we have explored in earlier chapters, values are shaped by many different influences. A health professional student absorbs professional values through role modelling and what has been called the hidden curriculum as previously mentioned in chapter 1.

Health professionals as educators

Health professionals are role models in the workplace whether they have an explicit contract to teach or not. So we could say that health professionals are constantly affecting learning. Junior professionals and students watch what is going on around them. Indeed students frequently do not have specific tasks other than observation in their early clinical rotations. Before entering the clinical environment, students will most likely have been taught about appropriate professional behaviour at university, during what are commonly referred to as personal and professional development (PPD) modules. They may have discussed values, but certainly will have been taught about ethics and ethical dilemmas. Hopefully, they will have been reflecting on their own values and whether these are appropriate for health care practice. Some students and junior staff reflect more than others. Some need to be facilitated to consider values and how their behaviour impacts not only on patient care but also on their peers and senior colleagues.

In personal and professional development programmes at university students are often given scenarios to discuss that have examples of 'good' and 'could do better' professional behaviour. When they have been on clinical placements, they may be asked to bring their own stories back to discuss in small groups. The professionalism of the clinicians they observe is rooted in their values. How professionals work with each other, how they communicate, what they say about other professionals, their interpersonal skills and their attitudes to team work are all on view and noticed by students and juniors.

Teamwork learning activities

A high proportion of our professional learning these days takes place in small groups and this is also true of prequalification training. While lectures are still common and cost-effective for transmitting information to a large number of people, small group teaching is often preferred as it fulfils more of the requirements for adult learning as described by Knowles (1990) (Box 15.2). This may be problem-based, case-based or task-based learning. A good group facilitator will help members understand that group processes are similar to team processes within working environments. The facilitator will also reflect back to the group how they are working together and what could be improved, relating this to clinical teams.

Box 15.2: Principles of adult learning

- Adults are autonomous and self-directed: they should be encouraged to set their own learning outcomes.
- Adults require facilitation rather than didactic teaching.
- Learning is best built on the learners' life experiences and existing knowledge; they should connect the learning activity to their current knowledge and skills.
- As adults are goal-orientated they want to know the purpose of the activity.
- They need to be motivated and understand the relevance of learning activities to their practice.
- Adults need to be stretched and receive constructive feedback.
- Adults need to be shown respect by the facilitator; they should be treated as equals in the learning environment.

Traditionally problem-based learning (PBL) and case-based learning (CBL) use problems and patient cases respectively as triggers for finding and working with information. However, educators now employ PBL and CBL in diverse ways and it is sometimes difficult to distinguish between them. One definition of PBL is 'learning that results from the process of working towards the understanding of a resolution of a problem. The problem is encountered first in the learning process' (Barrows & Tamblyn, 1980, p. 1). In contrast CBL has been defined as using a guided inquiry method, with defined learning outcomes, thus being more structured than PBL (Srinivasan et al., 2007). At university problems and cases can be written to meet not only science and clinical learning outcomes but ethical and professional outcomes, allowing discussion and reflection on challenging topics.

CBL is also referred to as case study teaching and case method learning. The Harvard Business School (HBS) adopted the case method across its curriculum in 1920 and it is still used today. Its website includes the following: 'when students are presented with a case, they place themselves in the role of the decision maker as they read through the situation and identify the problem they are faced with. The next step is to perform the necessary analysis – examining the causes and considering alternative courses of actions to come to a set of recommendations. To get the most out of cases, students read and reflect on the case, and then meet in learning teams before class to 'warm up' and discuss their findings with other classmates. In class – under the questioning and guidance of the professor – students probe underlying issues, compare different alternatives and finally, suggest courses of action in light of the organisation's objectives' (Harvard Business School, 2011). From this description it is obvious that this method of learning aims to mirror team working in practice and team meetings where decisions are made after considering options and, if appropriate, the patient's goals and expectations. HBS emphasises on its website the importance of values and expects students to share the community values of mutual respect, honesty, integrity and personal accountability.

Queen's University Centre for Teaching and Learning (Ontario, Canada) states that CBL 'focuses on the building of knowledge and the group works together to examine the case…the students collaboratively address problems from a perspective that requires analysis. Much of case-based learning involves learners striving to resolve questions that have no single right answer' (Queen's University 2011). Again the parallels with clinical work are obvious. However PBL and CBL often take place with uniprofessional groups, though as learning methods they are extremely suitable for IPE.

Depending on the learning outcomes, cases may be based on patient histories, but they can also focus on more specific issues relating to teamwork: cases of dysfunctional teams, or examples of adverse events arising from poor teamwork and communication. The scenarios in this book, for example, would make good triggers for discussion, and we may call this type of learning 'scenario-based learning'.

What is important for this type of learning is to define clearly what you expect the learners to learn – their learning outcomes. Too often these are forgotten, and participants may query the need to learn together, a process that may be difficult to organise logistically. Examples of frequently defined learning outcomes are listed in Box 15.3.

Box 15.3: Examples of learning outcomes for IPL activities (Thistlethwaite & Moran, 2010)

- Teamwork – *Knowledge of and skills for.*
- Roles and responsibilities – *Understanding of professional boundaries.*
- Communication – *Awareness of difference in professionals' language.*
- Learning/reflection – *Reflect critically on one's own relationship within a team.*
- The patient – *Demonstration of the patient's central role in interprofessional care.*
- Ethical/attitudes – *Understand one's own and others' stereotyping.*

Experiential learning

Reflection on group or team processes during learning is important. It helps to link the theories of teamwork and team function with the practical: what happens, or what should happen, in health care practice. Young health professional students, many straight from school, will have had limited experience of working in teams, though most will have been involved in sport (team based) or music (orchestra) and can draw on this in discussion. Experienced health professionals learning together bring a wealth of experience to share, and it is this experience that should form the basis of learning – building on what is already known. When working through a learning activity, the learning is more powerful if based on an example from a group participant. If the group is an actual health care team, the members can work through examples of current or past issues to discuss how they work together and how they might improve. Examples of this are significant event analysis as we have seen in Chapter 4, but teams should also work with examples of what has been done well and why.

We learn teamwork best by observation and practice, and reflection on that observation and practice, with feedback from others if possible. The theory behind such small group work is based on adult learning theory as described above, and here also known as experiential learning, i.e. learning through experience. The experiential learning cycle of Kolb (1993), derived from the earlier work of Lewin, explains the process (Box 15.4). While a learner may move round the cycle in a workplace, the process is also possible within a more structured team-based learning session. The observation and reflection is now no longer an individual process but also involves other team members, adding value to skill development (Elwyn et al., 2001).

Box 15.4: Kolb's experiential learning cycle in relation to teamwork

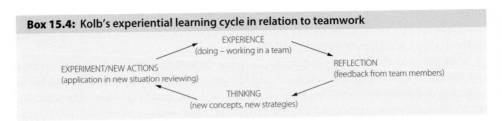

EXPERIENCE
(doing – working in a team)

REFLECTION
(feedback from team members)

THINKING
(new concepts, new strategies)

EXPERIMENT/NEW ACTIONS
(application in new situation reviewing)

Reflection point

How do you learn? How do you keep up-to-date? Do you prefer to learn by yourself or do you find a group learning process more rewarding? If in a group, would you choose a uniprofessional or interprofessional experience? Consider the process of reflection. How often do you reflect on your learning and how you have learnt?

There follow two examples of team-based learning activities. The first specifically focuses on values-based practice. The second is a case-based experiential learning session using role-play with the help of simulated patients.

One: A team training session for VBP

Rachel Meers is an experienced health care educator and interprofessional facilitator. Her own professional background is speech therapy but she has not worked as a clinician for 10 years. She has been asked to run a professional development session for the Sunshine Group Practice, a six doctor general practice in a deprived area on the outskirts of a major city.

Reflection point

What qualities, capabilities and values would you look for in an interprofessional facilitator for your team? Check these against Box 15.5. Do you think it is important that the facilitator is or has been a practising health professional? Why/why not?

The practice manager (Sunita Patel) and the education lead for the practice (Dr Lawrence Pope) would like a session on team work, particularly as the practice has several new members of staff and there is a feeling that communication and collegiality is not as strong as it could be. There has been some confusion as to which professional is responsible for what, and

Box 15.5: Capabilities required for interprofessional facilitation (adapted from Howkins & Bray, 2006)

- Generic facilitation skills.
- Reflective practice.
- Awareness of potential role conflicts.
- Interprofessional values.
- Open mindedness.
- Ability to challenge stereotyping.
- Ability to give constructive feedback.
- Acknowledgement of power and status issues within health care teams.

tension has been rather high. Rachel agrees to run an afternoon session for the wider team and there will be doctors, practice nurses, a nurse practitioner, practice counsellor, health visitor, one community nurse (more have found it difficult to free up time), receptionists, medical secretary and the practice manager. Lawrence and Sunita have briefed Rachel before the session and stressed how important they feel it is to have the team discuss how they are working together, problems they are facing and how things might improve. They also consider it important, as there are new staff, to re-visit the values of the practice and their commitment to the community.

Reflection point

Consider at this point what it is important to tell the staff about the session. They should have some idea about what the expected outcomes are but there should be flexibility for them to define their own problems and learning needs. If you were facilitating such a team learning activity yourself, what would you be considering about the process and what might be potential problems? As the facilitator what would you like to know about the practice, the team and the team members?

Looking at the make-up of the learning group and, without knowing much about this particular team's dynamics and values, or the individuals' values, Rachel will be wondering how comfortable various members may be in discussing what could be sensitive issues. Who are the new members of staff? Are they used to interprofessional education? Have the receptionists been involved in such activities before? Given that their 'bosses'/line manager are present, will they feel able to participate fully? How will the various professionals and administration staff learn and work together?

There are a number of ways that Rachel can run the session. Below is just one example. Rachel starts with introductions and asks participants for their expectations of the session (before this she will have been noticing who is sitting where, who is talking to whom etc). During the introductions she will observe who appears to be comfortable, who says a lot and who is quiet. She will then discuss the ground rules for the afternoon, asking for suggestions and again noticing who speaks first and longest. Ground rules may include: not interrupting colleagues when speaking, being respectful, turning off mobile phones, everyone to participate in discussions, confidentiality. Having considered what the group wants to achieve, she will adapt her plan to encompass this as well as to achieve the goals that Sunita and Lawrence have identified. She will list the proposed outcomes and check that there is agreement (Box 15.6 lists examples of possible outcomes). It is important that the outcomes for the session are clear to facilitate the learning process and help the participants know what they should achieve.

Box 15.6 – Examples of learning outcomes for a team-based learning activity

- An understanding of the term 'values'.
- An agreement on the practice's values.
- An exploration of how values might impact on our work.
- Exploration and discussion of team members' roles and responsibilities.
- Recommendations for any necessary changes in how we work together.

The first exercise will be a discussion of the practice's values – not forgetting that some of the staff are not directly employed by the practice but that they work with the same patients/clients. Rachel splits the participants into smaller groups ensuring that there is a mix of professions and roles within each group. Some of the more reticent participants may find it easier to contribute like this rather than have to address the whole room. The exercise is helped by trigger questions (Box 15.7). The groups then report back on the main points of their discussion to the larger group and Rachel ensures a consensus is reached. She also asks them what they have learnt from and about each other: did anything surprise them in the group discussion? Were there any differences in professional values?

Box 15.7: Trigger questions for the first activity

- What are values?
- What values do you/we bring to work? (personal and professional values).
- What are our team's values?
- Do we all agree with these values?
- Do we want to change these?
- Would these values fit with what our patients expect?

For the second activity of the afternoon Rachel asks people to think of one example of an incident in the practice, which exemplifies these values, and one incident where things could have been done better, where the values were not upheld. Just in case no-one volunteers any ideas, Rachel has been primed by Lawrence with two scenarios, but in fact the team, now warmed up, have several episodes they wish to discuss (Box 15.8). Rachel breaks them into mixed groups again with trigger questions (Box 15.9) to discuss and reminds them that this exercise is not about blame (though praise is fine) but about learning from experience: both good and not so good.

The incidents may appear minor, but they are the day-to-day issues that are rarely discussed at formal practice meetings, which are generally reserved for bigger problems relating to patient safety and adverse events.

In the de-brief several people mention that they are unclear about each other's roles. It is apparent that there has been some ill feeling when people are asked to do tasks that they do not feel are within their remit. Sometimes the tasks are beyond their scope of practice or capability; sometimes the tasks are 'beneath them'. This generates discussion about best use of people's skills but the consensus is that if necessary anyone should be prepared to do a 'lowly' task if it is necessary and there is no-one else to do it.

Box 15.8: Incidents for discussion

- **Incident 1:** Josie (practice nurse): I was running over 20 minutes late one morning. I called in my next patient and apologised for being late. He said: 'you are the first person in this practice who has ever said sorry for being late'. While punctuality is a value of course we cannot always be on time, but the receptionists should keep patients informed if we are running late, and I certainly think apologising doesn't hurt.
- **Incident 2:** Alice (GP): I have been seeing a 78 year old lady with multiple health problems for several months. Last week I saw she had developed a nasty ulcer on her right ankle. I haven't really had to deal with this sort of condition for a while but I remembered that Janice (one of the practice nurses) had been on a course recently about trauma, skin problems and new methods of treatment. We did a joint consultation with the patient and Janice really taught me a lot about the types of dressings I could use and follow-up care. I think working together like this is wonderful. [Janice adds that in her previous practice the doctors rarely asked her advice about anything and she finds it refreshing that the GPs here have no embarrassment about acknowledging that the nurses have a different and complementary skill set.]
- **Incident 3:** Joe (junior receptionist): I booked in a mother and her young son for an appointment with Janice, but I was told that it was more appropriate for the health visitor to deal with this type of problem. I don't really understand the distinction between what the different nurses do and would like some information for this and to give to patients so they can also decide who to see.
- **Incident 4:** Cheryl (medical secretary): I was in reception the other day and some of the staff (including a doctor, a nurse and a receptionist) were talking quite loudly about what they had got up to at the weekend. It's good to have a team spirit and be interested in one another, but what will the patients think? I didn't say anything because a GP was there and should know better.

Box 15.9: Trigger questions relating to incidents

- What happened?
- What have you/the team learnt from this incident?
- What values does this incident illustrate?
- How might things be done differently?
- How might the team improve following this incident and the discussion?
- What is the benefit of discussing incidents like this?

During the session Rachel ensures that she is meeting the agreed outcomes from the beginning of the afternoon. In the last half hour she revisits these and asks people whether their expectations have been met, what they have learnt, what has surprised them and what they might want to cover in another learning afternoon.

Two: Working with simulated patients

Simulated teamwork exercises are now an important part of both pre- and post-qualification health professional training. It is important to develop a scenario that is authentic, either based on an incident that has happened to students or participants within a clinical setting, or that is a common experience within health care settings that professionals need to be able to deal with.

Simulated patients are people, not necessarily professional actors but often so or recruited from amateur dramatics groups, who are trained to portray patients in a partially scripted scenario and who are able to respond authentically to the interactions they have with health professionals and/or students during learning activities (Box 15.10). They are able to give feedback in role to help learners enhance their skills and meet defined learning outcomes. Learning via simulation is a specialised method of experiential learning, allowing rehearsal, experiment, repetition and feedback, with both reflection on action and reflection in action.

> **Box 15.10:** Benefits of working with simulated patients (from Thistlethwaite & Ridgway, 2006)
>
> - Facilitator and learner have some control over environment.
> - Can plan specific learning outcomes by use of scenarios unlike opportunistic consultations in real clinical settings.
> - Ability to stop consultation/scenario at learning points if patient/learner distressed.
> - May re-run consultation/scenario to try different strategies.
> - Immediate feedback from patient or 'simulated professional'.
> - Feedback from group.
> - Learners can practise difficult consultations without risk of upsetting real patients.
> - Scenarios may be developed in response to learner's needs.

Rachel returns to the Sunshine Medical Practice 4 months after her previous visit. This time she is accompanied by two simulated patients: Roger and Bryony. Lawrence has briefed her a few weeks ago about some incidents at the surgery, which he would like to re-run with the staff so they will feel better equipped to deal with similar problems in the future. To avoid ruining the element of surprise with the scenarios the staff are only given some broad learning outcomes (Box 15.11) prior to the session without any details about the simulation that is about to unfold. They are aware, however, that the session will involve a simulation. There is also a discussion of the guidelines for giving feedback (see Chapter 3, Box 3.2, p. 120). Two camcorders are set up: one in reception and one in the treatment room.

> **Box 15.11:** Learning outcomes for the simulation
>
> - To enhance team skills in difficult situations.
> - To reflect on and gain a better understanding of one's own and one's colleagues' roles and responsibilities in difficult situations.
> - To discuss and improve communication between team members.
> - To reflect on the practice's values as reflected in the scenario and how these affected behaviour.

The scenario begins in the reception area (the surgery is closed for the afternoon as protected learning time). Everyone has been primed that the patients involved in the scenario are 'registered' patients of the practice. Joe and Christine, two of the receptionists, are behind the desk. Bryony is seated in view of reception. Roger enters the surgery – he is unshaven, scruffy and smells of alcohol. He demands to see a doctor straight away.

Christine offers an appointment for later that evening but Roger continues to demand he is seen 'now'. Joe leaves to find one of the health professionals. Meanwhile Bryony gives a moan, clutches her chest and falls to the floor. So the team have to deal with two 'emergencies', decide who does what and prioritise the tasks. While the GPs and two of the practice nurses treat Bryony, Sue (nurse practitioner) takes Roger into one of the consulting rooms with Joe (as a 'chaperone') and works through an interaction with Roger demanding a prescription for benzodiazepines.

The scenario runs for 20 minutes. Rachel then brings the team together and runs a feedback and debriefing session. They watch some of the recorded events. The ability to watch and reflect on what actually happened is an important part of the experience. 'I didn't realise I was just standing there doing nothing for so long' says Christine. Sue comments that she had really wanted to work with Bryony, whom she felt had greater medical need 'and was more deserving of my attention'. But having watched the play-back she now realises that her skills were put to very good use in dealing with Roger, who needed to be calmed down and taken out of the vicinity of the team working with Bryony. 'I was the best person at the time to interact with Roger. Division of labour within the team is important. I've lost my initial almost resentment of not being involved in the serious stuff of resuscitation, for which I'm trained, because I now know I also did a valuable job. We need to get our priorities right so we are all doing what is necessary.'

There are several areas in which the participants feel they could do better. In relation to managing Bryony's collapse, there was some confusion as to who should do what, and so they run through the event again. They also do this a third time with only one nurse and one receptionist (the receptionists have been trained in CPR). Sue does not feel she has handled her aggressive patient well and watches one of the experienced GPs interact with a very angry Roger. She then goes through the scenario again and feels more confident that she will defuse a similar situation more competently in the future.

There is a discussion about how the overall scenario and the teamwork reflect the values of the team. The team has never learned in this way before. They feel that this has complemented the discussion of the previous facilitated session, which focused more on talking together.

The evaluation of the session is very positive. The participants feel they have a better understanding of who should do what. Moreover the health professionals state that they now have a greater understanding of the skills and role of the receptionists as the frontline staff. What have they learnt about each other's values? The word that keeps being mentioned is 'professional': being calm, not flapping, ensuring the safety of both the team and the patients. Sue sums up the mood of the team: 'How can we work together if we don't learn and practise together? We have done our CPR training on manikins, but this added an extra dimension to practice and I now have a greater respect for my colleagues. Let's have more of this'. Joe comments that he had been angry himself at the way that Roger talked to both Bryony and Sue, and thought that there should be a practice policy that no-one under the influence of alcohol should be allowed to have a consultation. But he also realises that refusing to interact with Roger may have escalated the potential violence of the situation and that by involving another team member the situation could be defused. Keeping the team safe needs to be balanced against the needs of the patients; defusing a potentially dangerous situation by good interpersonal skills requires practice and experience.

Reflection point

Have you been involved in any teamwork simulation like that described? How do you think these activities help? What are the advantages and disadvantages of this type of education?

While working with simulated patients adds an extra dimension to learning, team members can work through interactions via role play to improve communication discuss and values.

For example, if we look at incident 4 in Box 15.8, Cheryl could role play giving feedback to the others in regard to their behaviour in reception. She may find this difficult in terms of the interaction with the doctor, but good facilitation will enhance her confidence.

Evaluation of learning

Reflection point

How would you evaluate a learning activity such as the one described? How do you know if the time was worthwhile for everyone, apart from by re-visiting the outcomes as described above?

Evaluation is important but can become tiresome especially if people do not feel that their evaluation is listened to or leads to change in the next education session. For example, if the participants say there is too much input by the facilitator and not enough discussion, this should be remedied.

There are two main categories of educational evaluation: process and outcome. Process evaluation, as it suggests, looks at the process of learning – how did the group interact; were the participants engaged; did most people contribute; did anyone appear to be drifting away? Such evaluation usually requires an observer, though an experienced facilitator may be able to fulfil both tasks if necessary. However, the facilitator may have unconscious bias and want to come across as having performed well (conflict of interest).

Outcome evaluation explores what participants have learnt during an activity and what effects that learning has on their knowledge, skills or behaviour. A commonly used framework for outcomes evaluation is that of Kirkpatrick (1994), which may be adapted for use with particular types of learning (Box 15.12).

Box 15.12: Different levels of evaluation (modified from Kirkpatrick, 1994)

- **Learner satisfaction:** Did the participants enjoy the session(s)? Were they satisfied with the content, delivery, pacing, scenarios, feedback and facilitators?
- **Learning outcomes:** Did the participants learn anything? Were they satisfied with the learning outcomes and were these met? Did they improve their skills or modify their attitudes?
- **Performance improvement:** Longer term evaluation. Did the learners change their behaviour as a result of the activity? Are they using their new skills in their workplace? Are they working better as a team?
- **Patient/health outcomes/organisational change:** These are the most difficult to evaluate and are therefore often left out. Has patient care improved as a consequence of the learning activity? Are things done differently in the workplace?

Communities of practice and their relevance for interprofessional learning

I would just like to mention here another term for the process of learning that has been applied to interprofessional activities. There is a great deal of commonality between them all with predominant foci of interaction, authenticity, experience and reflection.

'Situated learning theory' arises from the work of Lave & Wenger (1991) and their concept of communities of practice. Situated learning is the process by which we learn from our environments, interactions and work/social contexts, and fits well with the apprenticeship model so common within health professional education and development. From this theory we derive the process of 'legitimate peripheral participation' of those learners who are newcomers to the team, which Day (2006) has described clearly. The learners are legitimate as they are potential members of the health professional community (in general) and this particular team; they are peripheral as not yet fully involved in team activities; they participate in team activities and therefore learn about their profession, the team and their role within it by engaging in work.

All new team members are learners even though they may be fully qualified professionals. Not all are able to be peripheral as they orientate to their new team's values and practices, but this model helps us reflect on how new members learn from the role models within the team and cannot be expected to 'know everything' from day one.

Conclusion

A team does not come fully formed and functional into the workplace. Basing learning activities within the team, rather than professional development always being undertaken in uniprofessional groups, is an important part of team development. There is facilitated time and space to discuss values, roles, responsibilities and goals.

References

Barrows H and Tamblyn R. (1980). *Problem-based learning: an approach to medical education*. New York: Springer.

Day J. (2006). *Interprofessional working*. Cheltenham: Nelson Thornes.

Elwyn G, Greenhalgh T, Macfarlane F. (2001). *Groups. A guide to small group work in healthcare, management and research*. Abingdon: Radcliffe Medical Press.

Freeth D, Hammick M, Reeves S, Koppel I and Barr H. (2005). *Effective interprofessional education: development, delivery and evaluation*. Oxford: Blackwell Publishing.

Harvard Business School. (2011). Available at: http://www.hbs.edu/mba/academics/howthecasemethodworks.html (Accessed July 2011).

Howkins E and Bray J. (2006). *Preparing for interprofessional teaching. Theory and practice*. Abingdon: Radcliffe Medical Press.

Kirkpatrick DI. (1994). *Evaluating training programs: the four levels*. San Francisco: Berrett-Koehler.

Knowles MS. (1990) *The adult learner: a neglected species* (4th edition). Houston: Gulf Publishing.

Kolb DA. (1993). The process of experiential learning. In: Thorpe M, Edwards R and Hanson A (Eds). *Culture and processes of adult learning*. London: Routledge.

Lave J and Wenger E. (1991). *Situated learning – legitimate peripheral participation*. Cambridge: Cambridge University Press.

Queen's University. (2011). Available at: http://www.queensu.ca/ctl/goodpractice/case/index.html (Accessed July 2011).

Srinivasan M, Wilkes M, Stevenson F, Nguyen T and Slavin S. (2007). Comparing problem-based learning with case-based learning: effects of a major curricular shift at two institutions. *Academic Medicine*, **82**;74–82.

Thistlethwaite JE and Moran M. (2010). Learning outcomes for interprofessional education (IPE): literature review and synthesis. *Journal of Interprofessional Care*, **24**;503–513.

Thistlethwaite JE and Ridgway G. (2006). *Making it real. A practical guide to experiential learning*. Abingdon: Radcliffe Medical Press.

Afterword

Putting the final full stop at the end of the last sentence of a book causes conflicting emotions. It is great to finish a project that has involved a lot of time: reading and writing, reflecting and sometimes despairing. You have to finally let go, but I am already thinking how I could have written some parts differently, used other references, other scenarios – but there has to be an end sometime. Writing a book that focuses on teamwork is an odd process as a sole author. That is why I value the contributions and comments of colleagues, and I hope they add to the richness of the text.

My values are just that – my values. They have influenced the text, possibly in ways I am not completely conscious of. Readers will agree with some of what I have written – I hope not with all. Even the 'evidence' is open to question – I really doubt that anything can be wholly objective.

Being a health care professional is a privilege – people actually value our opinions, though they may not agree with them and may disregard them in their choice of treatment. Reciprocally we need to value our patients', clients' and colleagues' opinions, and by valuing them that means asking about them. All opinions are affected by values – just in the way we present information verbally and non-verbally we are sending out signals. Values-based practice is about awareness, openness and honesty. Teamwork is difficult especially in health care, when very diverse professionals come together with little time to gel. How often do we acknowledge that difficulty?

I hope you have found this book useful, perhaps challenging. You may have considered your own values and how they impact on your work and your team. You may have disagreed with some or a lot of what I have written – I am not expecting complete agreement: consider whether you disagree because our values conflict or because of our different professional backgrounds and/or experience. If we were working together, how would we cope and manage such disagreement?

I do think values change and adapt as we mature – if they don't I consider that is what turns us into 'grumpy old men and women', complaining about the state of the world, and how things aren't what they used to be. I don't mind getting old (that much) but I am trying to stave off the grumpiness.

Index